AF572513

Dementing Brain Disease in Old Age

3 Teaching and Training in Geriatric Medicine

W. Meier-Ruge, Basel (ed.)

Dementing Brain Disease in Old Age

KARGER 1993

Basel · Freiburg · Paris · London · NewYork · NewDelhi · Singapore · Tokyo · Sydney

The chapters by J. Ulrich, B. Fischer et al. and H.-P. Wirth were translated into English by S.C. Cooper, C.G. Kreeger and J.E. Smith.
Illustrations and graphical artwork by L. Chevrolet.

Library of Congress Cataloging-in-Publication Data
Dementing brain disease in old age / W. Meier-Ruge (ed.). –
(Teaching and training in geriatric medicine; 3)
Chapters by J. Ulrich, B. Fischer, et al., and H.-P. Wirth were translated into English.
Includes bibliographical references and index.
(alk. paper)
1. Senile dementia. I. Meier-Ruge, W. (William) II. Series.
[DNLM: 1. Dementia, Senile – diagnosis. 2. Dementia, Senile – physiopathology.
3. Dementia, Senile – therapy. W1 TE129L v.3]
RC524.D47 1993
618.97′68983–dc20
ISBN 3–8055–4478–2

Drug Dosage
The authors and the publisher have exerted every effort to ensure that drug selection and dosage set forth in this text are in accord with current recommendations and practice at the time of publication. However, in view of ongoing research, changes in government regulations, and the constant flow of information relating to drug therapy and drug reactions, the reader is urged to check the package insert for each drug for any change in indications and dosage and for added warnings and precautions. This is particularly important when the recommended agent is a new and/or infrequently employed drug.

Printed in Switzerland on acid-free paper by Friedrich Reinhardt AG, Basel
ISBN 3–8055–4478–2

Contents

Contributors

Prof. Dr. B. Fischer
Rehabilitationsklinik Klausenbach, D-W–7618 Nordrach-Klausenbach (FRG)

Dr. U. Fischer
Rehabilitationsklinik Klausenbach, D-W–7618 Nordrach-Klausenbach (FRG)

Prof. Dr. B. Forette
Groupe Hospitalier Sainte-Périne, 11, rue Chardon-Lagache,
F–75781 Paris Cedex 16 (France)

Dr. S. Lehrl
Abteilung für Medizinische Psychologie und Psychometrie der Psychiatrischen
Universitätsklinik Erlangen, Schwabachanlage 6–10, D-W–8520 Erlangen (FRG)

Dr. P. Slater
University of Manchester, Department of Physiological Sciences, Stopford Building,
Oxford Road, Manchester M13 9PT (England)

Prof. Dr. J. Ulrich
Department of Neuropathology, Institute of Pathology, University of Basel,
CH–4003 Basel (Switzerland)

Dr. H.-P. Wirth
Gastroenterologie, Medizinische Poliklinik, Universitätsspital, Rämistrasse 100,
CH–8091 Zürich (Switzerland)

Dr. H. Woelk
Rehabilitationsklinik Klausenbach, D-W–7618 Nordrach-Klausenbach (FRG)

Preface

This third volume of *Teaching and Training in Geriatric Medicine* deals with senile dementia. The book tries to inform the practitioner in a clear and easily understandable way about the recent findings in the pathogenesis and therapy of senile dementia. A basic knowledge about dementing brain disease and its course is also important for anyone charged with the care of a senile dementia patient in his or her family. The family will be aided in understanding the conduct of the patient and in coping with his or here care.

Teaching and Training in Geriatric Medicine was designed as a series of books giving the busy practitioner and clinician simple information about the present state of knowledge in geriatric medicine. The didactic form in which the books are presented gives each page its own headline. The left-hand page contains a short, simple text. Each text page ends with a blue-marked summary containing the essential points. The right-hand page presents figures, photographs, diagrams, questionnaires etc. with an accompanying legend. In this way the busy reader can obtain at least 50% of the information from the headlines, the summaries and the illustrations. An extensive index helps to locate subjects of particular interest.

The editor thanks the staff of S. Karger, Medical Book Publishers, for their cooperation in producing this book. They always supported the work with great effort and patience.

W. Meier-Ruge
Associate Professor of Pathology
Division of Gerontologic Brain Research
Department of Pathology
University of Basel

The Neuropathology of Senile Dementia

J. Ulrich

What Is 'Organic Dementia'?

All patients with diffusely distributed degenerative brain changes visible under the microscope or with the naked eye show similar clinical signs such as impairment of intellect and memory. Demonstration of this was a valuable scientific contribution of psychiatry at the beginning of the century. This finding made it possible to differentiate 'organic mental diseases' (organic psychoses) from 'endogenous' psychoses (schizophrenia and manic depressive psychosis) and from 'reactive' mental disorders. This section will describe the microscopic neuropathological changes and correlate them with the neurological and psychiatric symptoms.

The most common cause of organic dementia is Alzheimer's disease, followed by multi-infarct dementia and combinations of the two. In addition, Parkinson's disease may give rise to psycho-organic symptoms (= mild dementia). Less frequent causes are encephalitis, communicating hydrocephalus, Pick's 'circumscribed brain atrophy' and the recently described form of dementia characterized by argyrophilic granules (i.e. granules which can be visualized with silver salts). Dementia can doubtless also result from hypoxic episodes due to circulatory collapse, poisoning and deficiency diseases. In Europe and the USA the sequelae of severe chronic alcohol abuse (e.g. Korsakoff's syndrome) are among the dementias with a toxic causation.

In seeking to make a differential diagnosis the clinician is frequently faced with the problem of distinguishing organic dementias, on the one hand, from psychic changes resulting from localized brain damage and, on the other hand, from depression. Since both depression as well as tumours are amenable to treatment, it is vital that the differential diagnosis of dementia should be undertaken with great care using all available diagnostic aids.

Organic dementia results from diffuse morphological degenerative brain disease. The differential diagnosis from depression and mental disturbances due to brain tumours is of great practical importance.

Diffuse brain atrophy in Alzheimer's disease

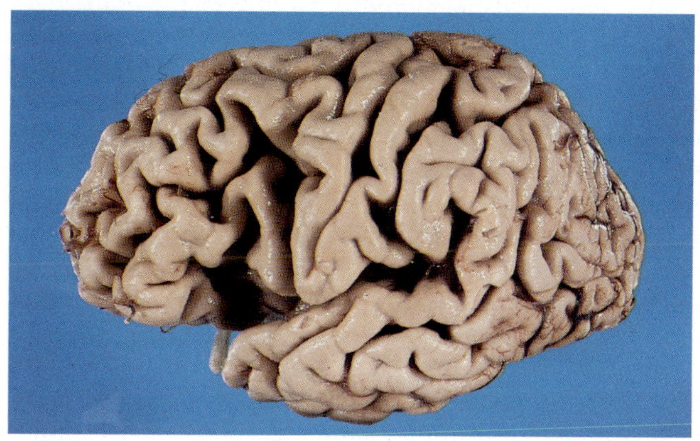

The characteristic morphological substrate of organic dementia is thc wide sulci which are readily visible to the naked eye.

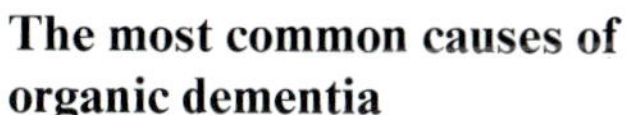

The most common causes of organic dementia

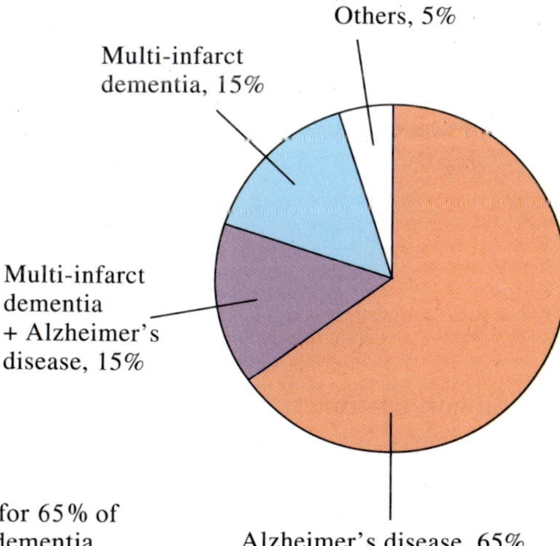

Alzheimer's disease which accounts for 65% of cases is the most common cause of dementia.

A Little Bit of Neurobiology and Neuromorphology

General Structural Principles of the Central Nervous System

For an easier understanding of specific brain changes in Alzheimer's disease, let us first examine some basic neuro-anatomical features of the brain.

The central nervous system consists of neurons (nerve cells) and glia cells. Here we shall confine ourselves to a description of the *neurons.* These consist of a cell body (pericaryon) and two types of processes: dendrites and axons. The axons are usually long (often several centimetres) and thin (usually less than 10 μm). The dendrites are thick (their proximal sections are up to 20 μm thick) and relatively short (less than 1 mm). The neurons are in contact with each other via synapses. Synapses are specially differentiated interneuronal zones of contact at the cell surface. They are recognizable under the electron microscope by their osmiophilia, which is due to presynaptic and postsynaptic thickening of the membrane. The surface area of a synapse measures about 0.1 μm^2.

In one of the two cell processes of two nerve cells meeting at the *synapse* there are fine vesicles. These contain a transmitter substance, a neurotransmitter. When an excitatory impulse reaches the presynaptic process, a small quantity of neurotransmitter is released into the synaptic cleft. The latter is located at specialized sections of the postsynaptic process and has receptors for the neurotransmitter. Postsynaptic binding of neurotransmitter leads to excitation of the postsynaptic neuron.

As a rule the presynaptic half of the synapse is on an axon, and the postsynaptic part on the pericaryon or in the dendrite. We therefore speak of axosomatic and axodendritic synapses. However other combinations are also found, e.g. axoaxonal and dendrodendritic synapses.

The feltwork of neuronal processes in the grey matter of the brain is known as the *neuropil.*

Central nervous function is accomplished by neurons (nerve cells) which are interconnected by synapses. The feltwork of neuronal and glia cell processes outside the neuronal and glia cell bodies is called the neuropil. Neurons communicate with the aid of chemical transmitter substances (neurotransmitters) which are transferred at specialized zones of contact (synapses).

The interconnection of nerve cells

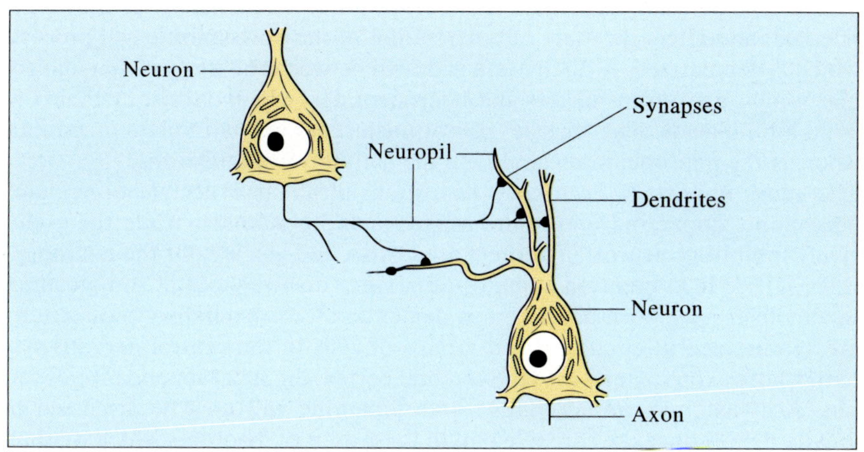

Nerve cells (neurons) are interconnected by means of synapses and communicate by release of chemical transmitter substances, known as neurotransmitters [after A. Probst].

Neuropil and synapses (approximately × 10,000)

a = Dendrite
s = Synapse,
presynaptic process

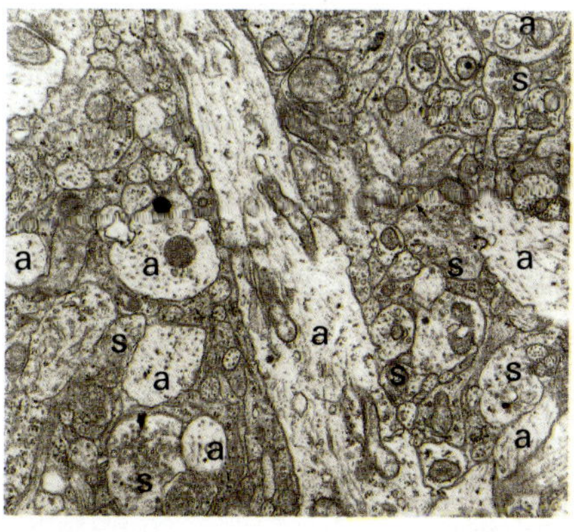

Electron microscopy affords an insight into the 'jigsaw puzzle'-like feltwork of the neuropil with synapses and dendrites.

A Little Bit of Neurochemistry

Some Neurotransmitters of the Brain

As already mentioned, when the wave of electrical depolarization reaches the presynaptic neuronal process, a transmitter substance, a neurotransmitter, is released, and alters the state of polarization of the postsynaptic cell process, which is depolarized. A distinction is drawn between the 'classic', low-molecular weight neurotransmitters and neuropeptides, which consist of chains of 3–20 amino-acids. The 'classic' neurotransmitters may stimulate or inhibit, whereas the neuropeptides modulate the activity of the neurons.

The most important excitatory neurotransmitters are acetylcholine, noradrenaline, dopamine, serotonin, aspartate and glutamate, while the exclusively inhibitory neurotransmitters are GABA and glycine. Of the neuropeptides suffice it to mention somatostatin, since disturbances of somatostatin metabolism have been described in dementia. Some excitatory transmitters are synthesized in circumscribed groups of cells in the central nervous system, whose axons extend into the cerebral cortex, the striatum and hippocampus. Acetylcholine, noradrenaline and dopamine will now be discussed in greater detail, since they are relevant to the groups of disorders which we shall be dealing with.

Acetylcholine is formed in large neurons at the base of the frontal lobe of the brain. The axons from these neurons run to the neopallium (the cerebral cortex) and to the hippocampus (also called Ammon's horn because of its shape).

Noradrenaline is produced in the locus coeruleus, a bluish pigmented nucleus in the lateral angle of the floor of the fourth ventricle. The axons from this small nucleus (which measures about $11 \times 1 \times 1$ mm) pass to every part of the central nervous system. The connections with the cerebral cortex are of particular interest to us.

Dopamine is produced by neurons of the substantia nigra. Their axons run mainly to the striatum, and the distribution of this neurotransmitter is much more narrowly circumscribed than that of the other neurotransmitters.

Groups of neurons which synthesize acetylcholine, serotonin, dopamine and noradrenaline send their axons to the telencephalon (end-brain), particularly to the cerebral cortex. They are of importance in connection with the pathogenesis of dementia.

Cholinergic and noradrenergic projection systems

Cholinergic system

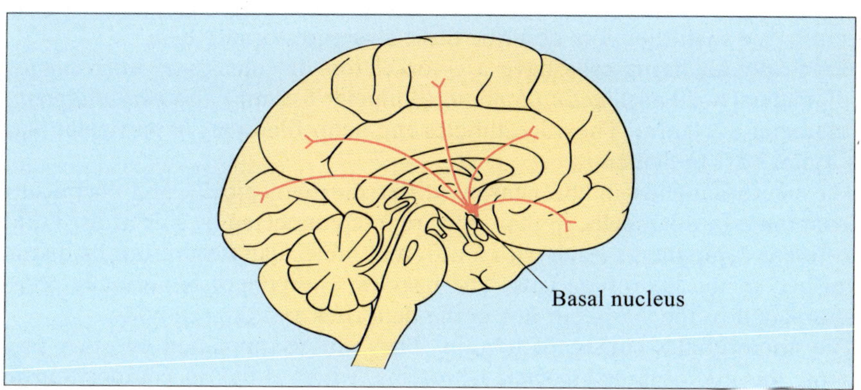

Axons from the basal nucleus run in large numbers to the cerebral cortex and subserve an important function in cognitive (mental) performance.

Noradrenergic system

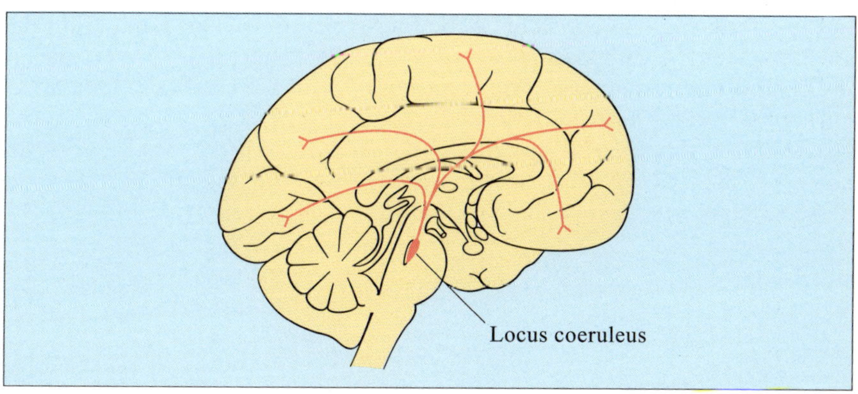

Nerve fibres from the locus coeruleus run to almost every part of the brain and stimulate or modulate nerve cells.

A Little Bit of Neurocytology

The Cytoskeleton and Its Importance for Senile Dementia

Surprisingly enough the most striking changes in dementia do not affect those components of the nerve cells which are known to be concerned with their function, such as the synapse and cell membranes. The changes occur in the filamentous structures (the cytoskeleton) within the nerve cells and their processes. We shall therefore describe these structures briefly here.
Practically all living cells have a cytoskeleton. It consists of *microtubules* (diameter 16–20 nm), *actin filaments* (diameter 6–8 nm) and *neurofilaments* (diameter 8–10 nm). The microtubules and neurofilaments in particular play a major part in dementia.
The neurofilaments of the neurons differ morphologically and chemically from those of other cells, in that they are interconnected by side arms. Three different components, each with a different molecular weight, can be distinguished in the neurofilaments. The heaviest component is normally phosphorylated in the axon, but not in the dendrites and the cell body.
The microtubules consist of tubulin. They are accompanied by other proteins, the microtubule-associated proteins, which differ in composition in different parts of the cell. Phosphorylated microtubule-associated tau protein is the form mainly found in the axon.

The most striking microscopic findings in dementia are those affecting the cytoskeleton. In normal neurons many proteins of the axonal cytoskeleton are phosphorylated, whereas those of the cell body and dendrites are not.

Axon showing microtubules and neurofilaments
(approximately × 50,000)

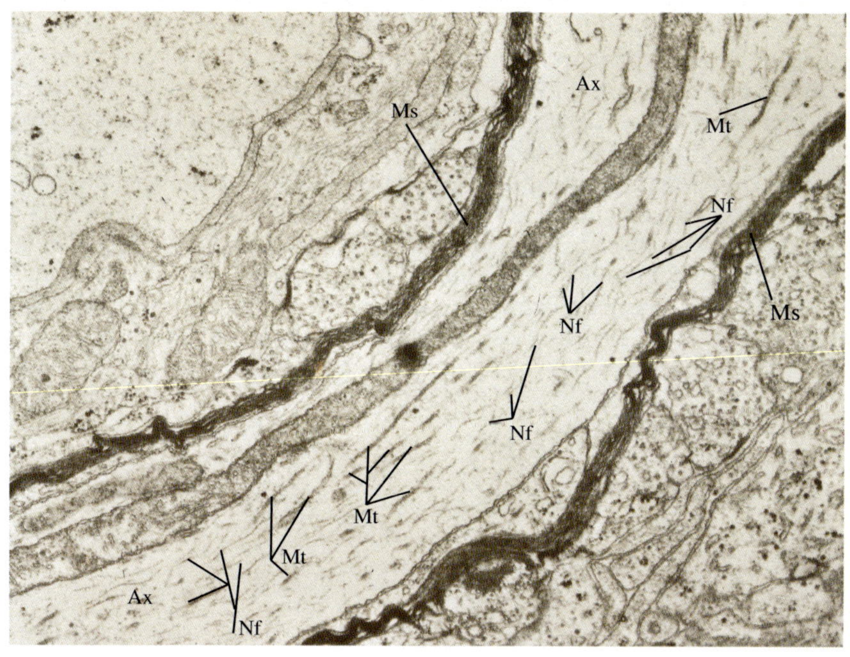

Ax = Axon
Nf = Neurofilament
Mt = Microtubules
Ms = Myelin sheath

The figure shows the submicroscopic organization of an axon where it leaves the nerve cell; the various structural elements of the axon may be seen.

Alzheimer's Disease and Senile Dementia

Alzheimer's disease is a brain disorder characterized by *senile plaques* and *Alzheimer's neurofibrillary change.* It is common in elderly people, but also occurs occasionally in the presenium (from about the age of 50 onwards). Since the female patient first described by Alzheimer developed dementia at the age of 52 years, the term Alzheimer's disease was for many years reserved for presenile cases (early form of the disease). In elderly patients, the term senile dementia of the Alzheimer type was introduced. From the morphological standpoint this is, we believe, an artificial distinction, and we therefore use the term Alzheimer's disease for all cases of dementia showing the same structural brain changes.

Since Alzheimer's disease is not necessarily accompanied by cerebral atrophy, and since furthermore other cerebral disorders leading to dementia may be accompanied by cerebral atrophy, radiographic evidence of cerebral atrophy does not suffice to distinguish the various diseases of the brain.

The most common cause of organic dementia is Alzheimer's disease, which can be diagnosed histologically from the presence of senile plaques and Alzheimer's neurofibrillary change. As a rule the diagnosis is reached by neuropathological examination of the brain at autopsy.

Diagram showing the typical histological changes in Alzheimer's disease

Senile plaques

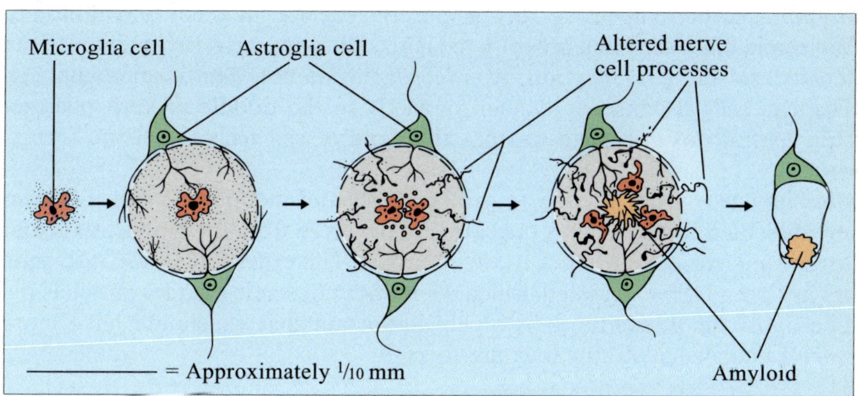

From left to right the process whereby the plaques probably develop. In recent years it has been demonstrated that the formation of a senile plaque is ushered in by the appearance of a phagocytic microglia cell. At a later stage amyloid accumulates at the centre of the plaque [after A. Probst].

Nerve cell with a normal cytoskeleton and a nerve cell containing Alzheimer neurofibrils

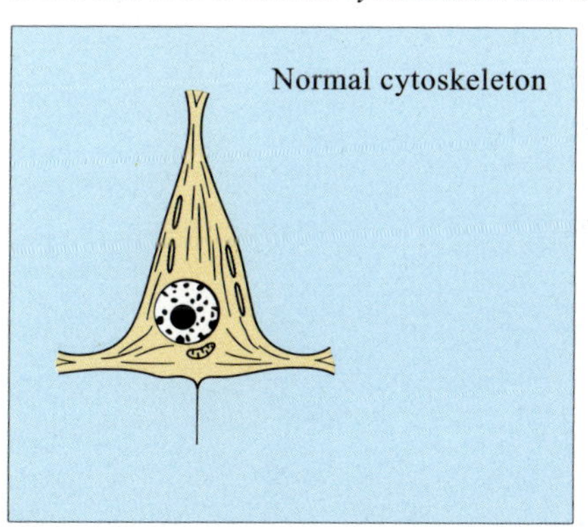

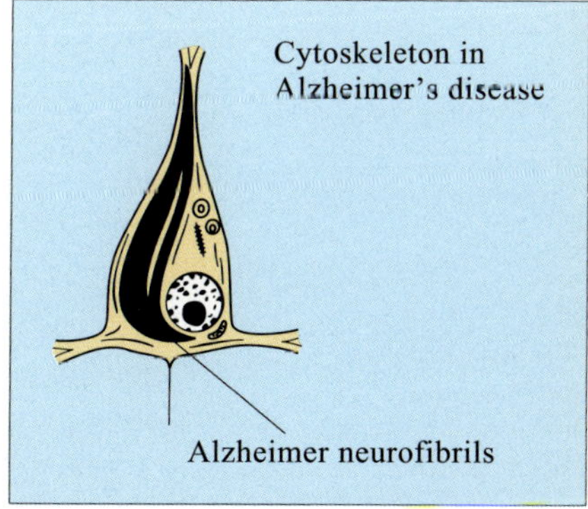

Nerve cells developing Alzheimer's neurofibrillary changes have apparently lost their function and if present in large numbers are typical of senile dementia (Alzheimer's disease).

What Occurs When Senile Plaques Form in the Grey Matter?

Senile plaques are spherical components of altered neuropil, the feltwork of nerve cell processes which make up the grey matter of the brain. They are about 1/10 of a millimetre in diameter. The plaques consist for the most part of amyloid, altered neuronal processes and glial cells, whose function and origin has hitherto been regarded as purely 'reactive'. It is not uncommon to find senile plaques which are only recognizable from the rather greater tissue density and the glial reaction. It is interesting to note that a microglial cell (Hortega cell) is consistently found exactly in the middle of such plaques. This central position suggests that this type of cell triggers plaque formation.

Microglia are closely related to macrophages and monocytes, and it is conceivable, therefore, that they migrate into the brain from the bloodstream and initiate a destructive process in the neuropil. The exact role of the microglia has not been fully elucidated. Since the number of senile plaques parallels the severity of the dementia, it is highly important that we should have more precise knowledge of how they are formed.

Senile plaques are altered areas of the grey matter. The microglia play an important but not yet fully elucidated part in their formation.

The structure of the senile plaque

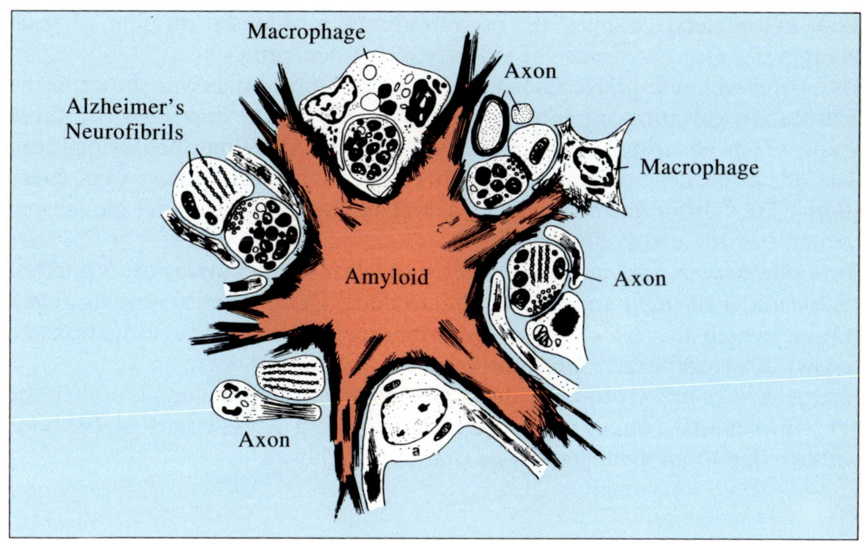

Diagram of a senile plaque [after A. Probst].

Early stages in the development of a senile plaque

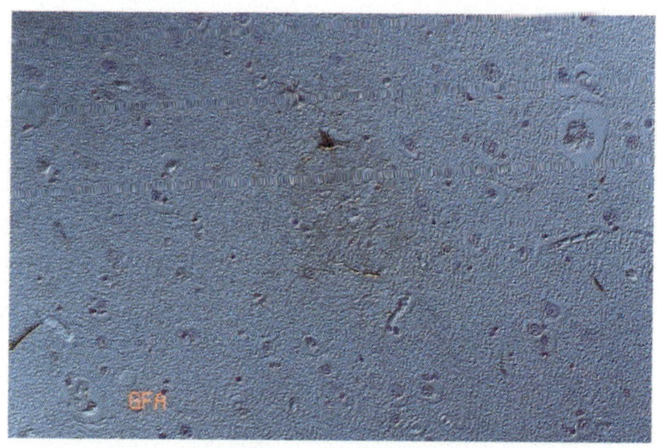

In this figure the glial fibrillar protein is stained, thus revealing the finest ramifications of the astrocytes. The plaque evidently emits a powerful stimulus promoting formation of glial fibrils.

Alzheimer's Neurofibrillary Change, Granulovacuolar Degeneration and Hirano Bodies as Indicators of the Severity of Alzheimer's Disease

The cytoskeletal changes include Alzheimer's neurofibrillary change, granulovacuolar degeneration and formation of Hirano bodies. The reason why these cytoskeletal changes are of importance is that the number of such changes parallels the degree of severity of the dementia.

The *Alzheimer neurofibril* (its light microscopic appearance was shown in the neurobiological introduction) is definitely the most important of these changes. The electron microscope reveals that the Alzheimer neurofibril consists of paired helical filaments, each 10 nm thick, which cross over every 80 nm. They differ morphologically as well as chemically from all the normal elements of the cytoskeleton.

Granulovacuolar degeneration consists of clear intracytoplasmic vacuoles, visible under the light and electron microscope. Each vacuole contains a dark granule which has been shown by immunocytochemical investigations to consist of neurofilament proteins.

Hirano bodies are eosinophil intracytoplasmic structures visible under the light microscope, whose ultrastructure displays a chess-board or fishbone pattern, due to an arrangement of filaments in layers.

The neurons of patients with Alzheimer's disease display various cytoskeletal changes, the most important being Alzheimer's neurofibrillary change.

Less common cytoskeletal changes in Alzheimer's disease

Light microscopy

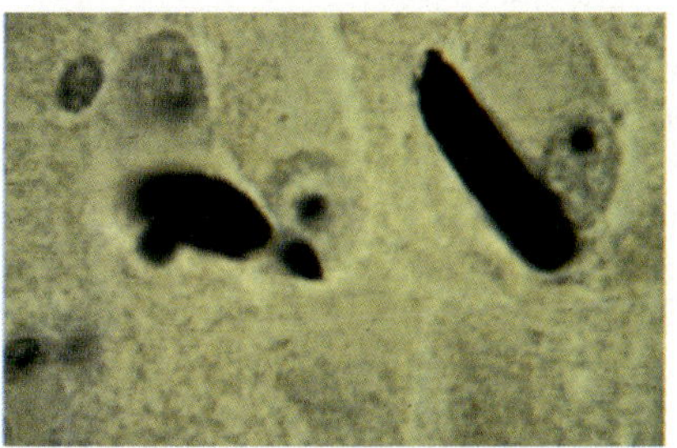

Hirano bodies

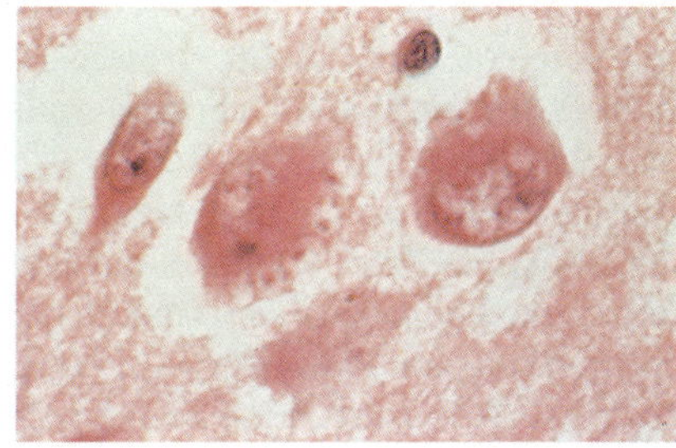

Granulovacuolar degeneration

The number of cells with Hirano bodies and/or granulovacuolar degeneration, together with those containing Alzheimer fibrils, is a measure of the degree of severity of Alzheimer's disease.

Electron microscopy

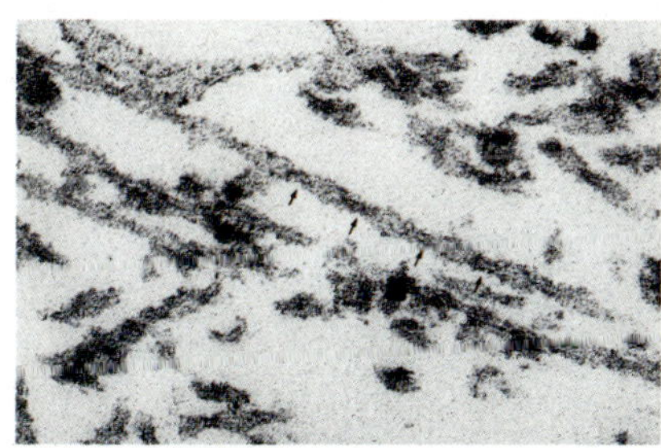

Alzheimer fibrils
(paired helical filaments) with periodically recurring constrictions (arrows, distance 80 nm)

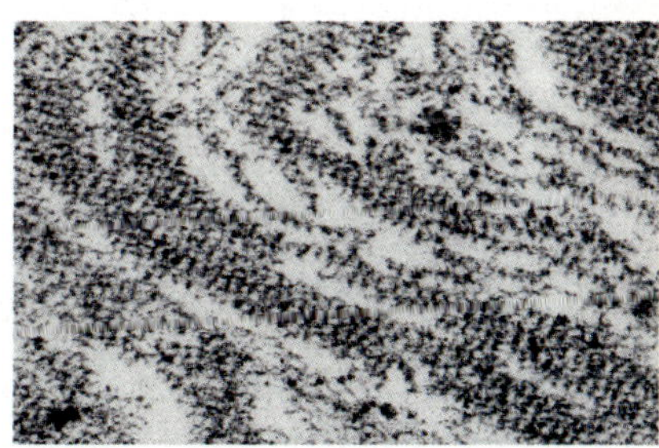

Components of a Hirano body

The electron microscopic appearance of Alzheimer neurofibrillary change is just as characteristic as that of the Hirano bodies. Although we know a great deal about the structure of the neurofibrils, the mechanisms whereby they are formed have yet to be elucidated.

The Application of Enzyme Histochemistry and Immunohistology to the Cytoskeleton

In the last 10 years immunohistological methods have considerably widened our knowledge of the cytoskeletal changes occurring in Alzheimer's disease. For example, cytoskeletal proteins can now be visualized and located routinely in paraffin wax sections. Such techniques have revealed, for example, that some neurofilament proteins in the axon contain phosphate groups, whereas the equivalent neurofilament proteins in the normal pericaryon do not.

Immunocytochemical investigations using antibodies to phosphorylated and non-phosphorylated cytoskeletal proteins have shown that cells which have undergone neurofibrillary change contain phosphorylated proteins. Thus the changed neuron contains cytoskeletal proteins which are normally present in the axon. It is interesting to note that the same proteins also occur in Pick bodies – the nerve cell inclusions occurring in Pick's disease – although these bodies differ completely in ultrastructure from Alzheimer neurofibrils. Since both diseases are associated clinically with dementia, there are strong grounds for suspecting that the abnormal localization of phosphorylated proteins plays a part in the development of the disorder.

Cell counts have shown that the presence of Alzheimer neurofibrils leads to the death of the nerve cells affected. After the death of the cell, the Alzheimer neurofibrils come to lie outside the cell, and trigger a powerful astrocytic reaction accompanied by a glial fibrillary reaction. Such features are known as neuron 'tombstones'. Some clinical symptoms of dementia may be due to cell death.

New immunohistochemical methods permit visualization and localization of minute concentrations of altered proteins in microscopic sections. Such techniques have revealed that in Alzheimer's disease certain phosphorylated proteins which normally occur only in the axon can also be demonstrated in the neuronal cell body.

Application of immunohistology in organic dementia

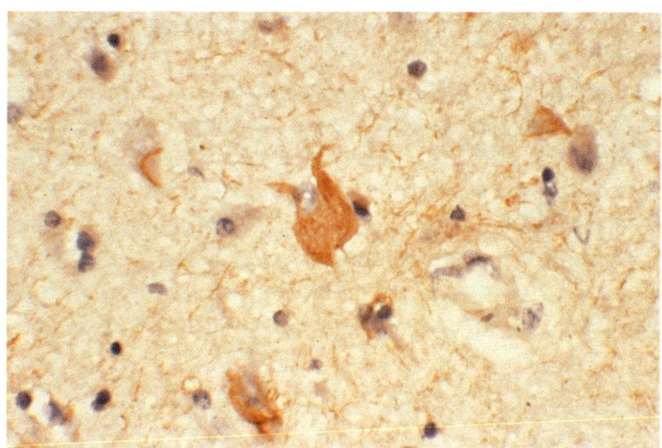

Visualization of Alzheimer fibrils with a monoclonal antibody to phosphorylated neurofilament proteins.

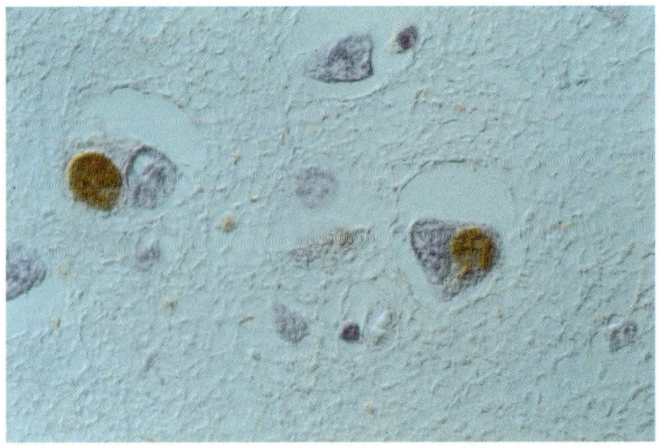

Visualization of Pick bodies with the same specific antibody used for Alzheimer fibrils. Immunohistochemistry has shown that the cell bodies of nerve cells contain proteins which normally only occur in the axons.

Correlation between the Clinical Signs and Symptoms and the Pathological Features of Alzheimer's disease

In the investigation of Alzheimer's disease it is important to seek correlations between the clinical, morphological and chemical findings. The first attempts to correlate the clinical signs and symptoms with the morphological findings date back almost 30 years.

Patients from geriatric hospitals were systematically examined using batteries of psychological tests which permitted quantification of their mental performance. On the death of these patients an autopsy was carried out and neurofibrillary changes in the brain were counted per brain section and brain region. These findings were then correlated with the psychological test results. The severity of dementia paralleled the severity of the pathological changes. Similar correlations with transmitter deficits were sought in later studies. All the findings paralleled the degree of severity of the dementia.

The greater the number of senile plaques, Alzheimer neurofibrils, other neuronal cytoskeletal changes and neurotransmitter deficits that are present, the more severe the dementia.

Diagram illustrating some features of cerebral disorders associated with dementia

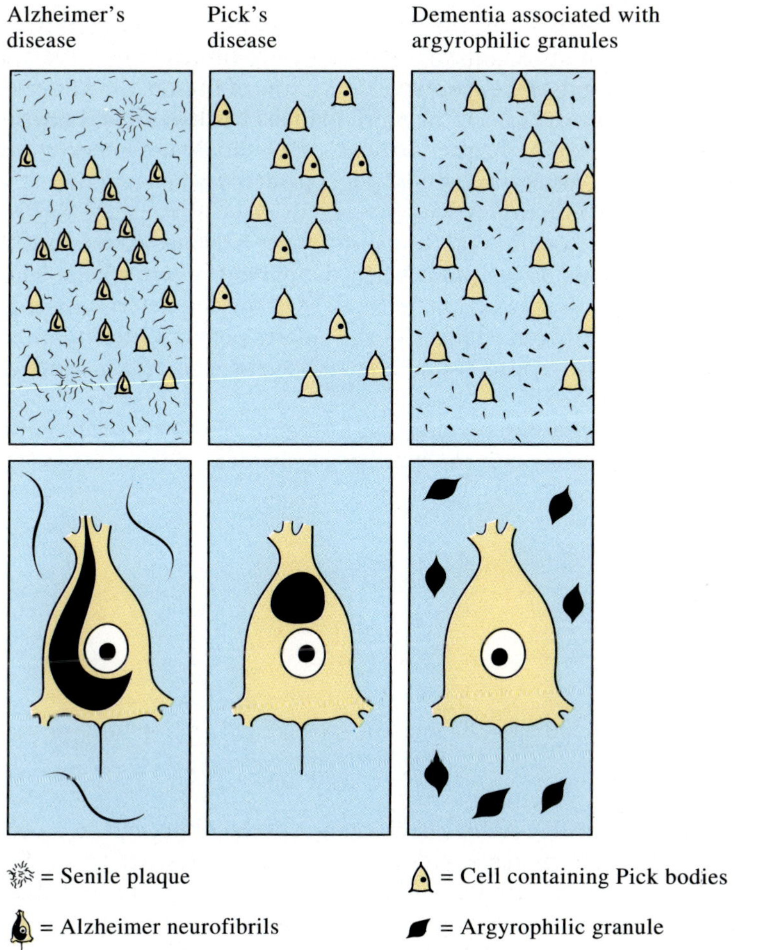

The figures show that dementia need not necessarily be associated with the features of Alzheimer's disease, although that is the case in 65% of age-related dementia cases. Drawing reproduced with permission of H. and E. Braak.

Normal Aging and Alzheimer's Disease

From the age of 65 years onwards the human brain shows a slight decrease in weight. Moreover, the brains of nearly all elderly people display isolated senile plaques and Alzheimer's neurofibrillary change.

From the correlations between the morphological and the psychological findings, it may be regarded as established that dementia results from development of senile plaques and Alzheimer fibrils. As a rule of thumb, the presence of numerous senile plaques (some 5 or more plaques per high-power microscopic field) is indicative of Alzheimer's disease. This should not be taken too literally, since practical aspects must also be considered when arriving at a diagnosis of Alzheimer's disease.

It is a useful expedient to define the transition from harmless senile forgetfulness to senile dementia as the point when the patient requires help. This transition need not necessarily be precipitated by a sudden deterioration in the brain, but may result from changes in the elderly person's life situation, such as a change of domicile, admission to an old person's home, the death of a close relative, etc.

It is interesting to note that the memory performance of elderly people who are not demented correlates with the number of plaques.

Nearly all old people display Alzheimer's change in the brain, but to a considerably less extent than patients with dementia. The difference between a normal aged brain and the brain of an old patient with dementia is not absolute. Manifestation of dementia is not solely determined by the typical brain lesions of Alzheimer's disease. Often dementia, for which the way has been prepared by structural brain changes, is triggered by sudden changes in the accustomed environment of the elderly person (admission to an old person's home, change of domicile, death of a close relative, etc.).

Alzheimer's disease is characterized by the extent of the Alzheimer changes

Normal aging

Senile dementia

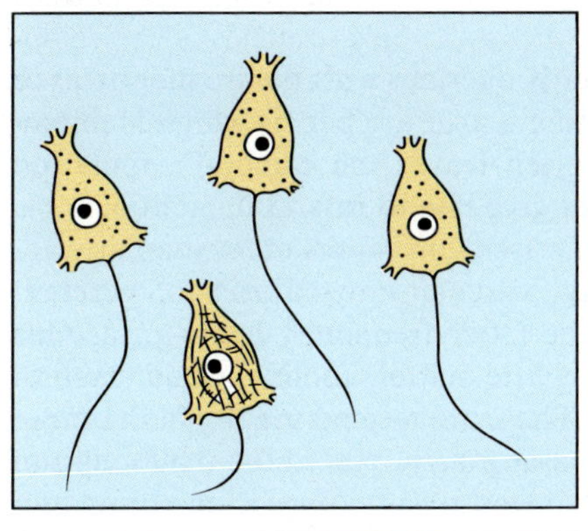

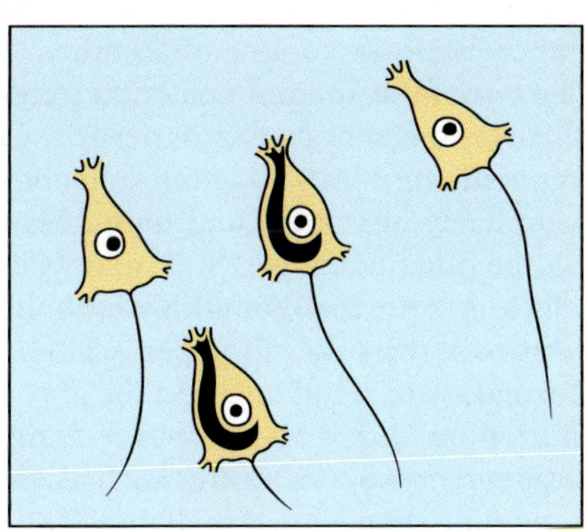

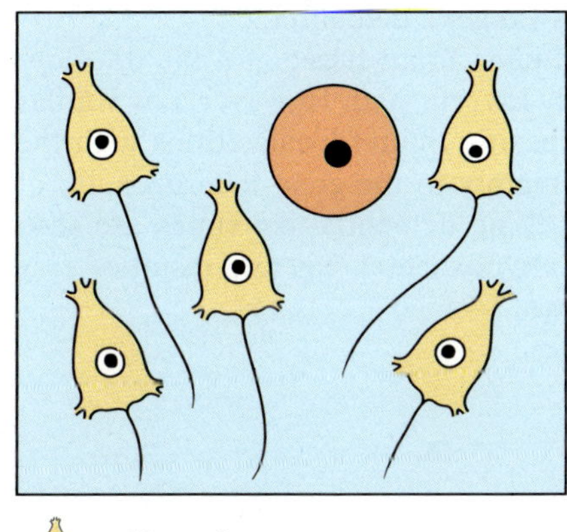

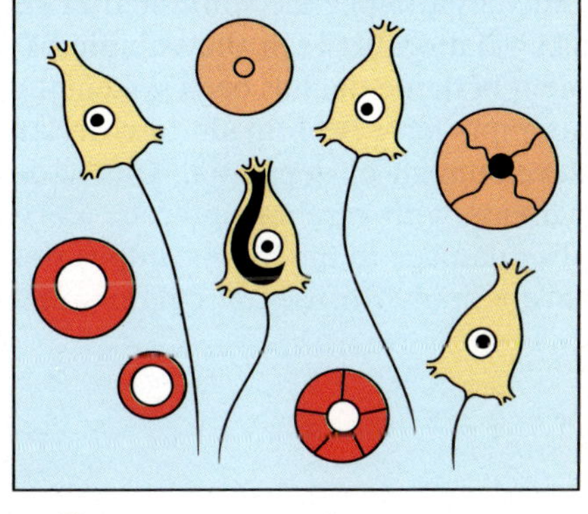

 = Normal neuron

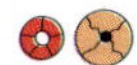 = Typical types of senile plaques

 = Neuron showing Alzheimer's change

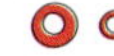 = Blood vessels

This diagram seeks to convey the impression obtained on examining brain sections from a patient with senile dementia (Alzheimer's disease) (right) with those obtained on examining the brain of a person of the same age who was not suffering from dementia (left). Whether a patient develops Alzheimer's disease or not depends upon the number of senile plaques and Alzheimer's neurofibrillary changes.

Multi-Infarct Dementia

As the name implies, multi-infarct dementia results from numerous, usually very small infarcts. In exceptional instances a *few* large infarcts may give rise to a similar form of dementia. Systematic evaluation of the data has shown that dementia inevitably ensues once the volume of destroyed brain substance attains a volume of 50 ml.

The term multi-infarct dementia frequently overlaps with the frequently used older term cerebral arteriosclerosis. Cerebral arteriosclerosis which is in fact frequent *may* lead to infarction, but often leaves the cerebral circulation completely unscathed and then does not give rise to infarct dementia.

On the other hand, cerebral infarcts can arise from causes other than arteriosclerosis, principally multiple embolisms, vascular amyloidosis and cerebral arteriosclerosis due to hypertension. The latter frequently leads to lacunae (formation of small holes) in the grey or white matter, i.e. tiny round cerebral infarctions with a diameter of 3–5 mm. These are located mainly in the inner large cerebral nerve centres such as the basal ganglia, and in the thalamus and pons. The same vascular changes can also lead to softenings in the brain and demyelination of the white matter (Binswanger's dementia).

The relation between the volume of softened brain tissue and the development of dementia has been systematically investigated. However, few similar attempts have been made to correlate specific infarct localizations with the development of dementia. This is due mainly to the great heterogeneity of patients with cerebral infarcts. Very striking dementia-like states are seen after damage to the hippocampus due to hypoxaemia, e.g. as a result of very severe bradycardia or circulatory collapse.

The term multi-infarct dementia fits the pathogenetic mechanism of this dementia syndrome more accurately than the term cerebral arteriosclerosis, especially as destruction of brain tissue due to small infarcts is the decisive factor in the development of multi-infarct dementia.

Status lacunaris of the thalamus as a cause of multi-infarct dementia

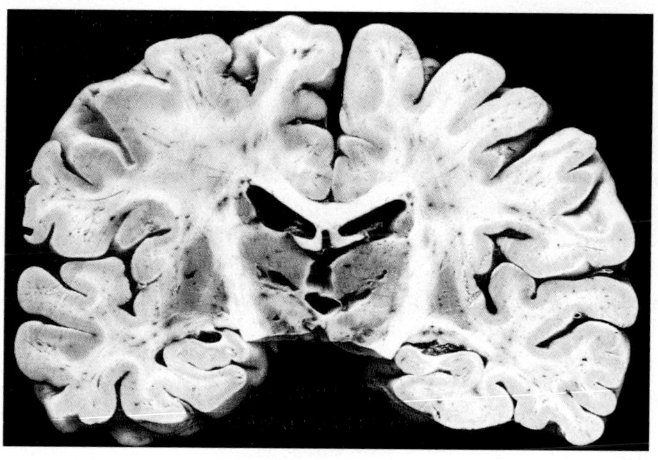

In multi-infarct dementia the thalamus frequently displays small holes or lacunae. They are what is left when small infarcts have healed. Status lacunaris is only one of the possible morphological pictures seen in multi-infarct dementia.

Parkinson's Disease

Dementia may also develop in Parkinson's disease. For this reason we shall examine briefly the morphology of this disorder. The prominent features are degeneration of the substantia nigra (a nucleus comprising nerve cells containing black pigment). The pigmented nerve cells die and their pigment escapes from the nerve cells and is taken up by macrophages of the other brain tissue.

Characteritic of Parkinson's disease is the presence of inclusion bodies in neurons. These bodies consist of a filamentous substance and have a concentric layered structure (Lewy bodies). They too contain phosphorylated components of the normal cytoskeleton. These inclusion bodies (Lewy bodies) are found in various nuclei in the brainstem and sometimes also in the sympathetic trunk. The neurotransmitters of most of the nuclei so affected are catecholamines, but some (especially the basal nucleus) also employ acetylcholine as neurotransmitter.

This latter observation is of much interest, since cholinergic deficits also occur in Alzheimer's disease. It has therefore been postulated that the parkinsonian patients who develop dementia are those whose cholinergic basal nucleus is also affected. No systematic studies have as yet been carried out to verify whether this is the case.

Dementia sometimes develops in Parkinson's disease. It may be attributed to involvement of the cholinergic basal nucleus.

Brain pathology in Parkinson's disease

Macroscopic appearance of the substantia nigra

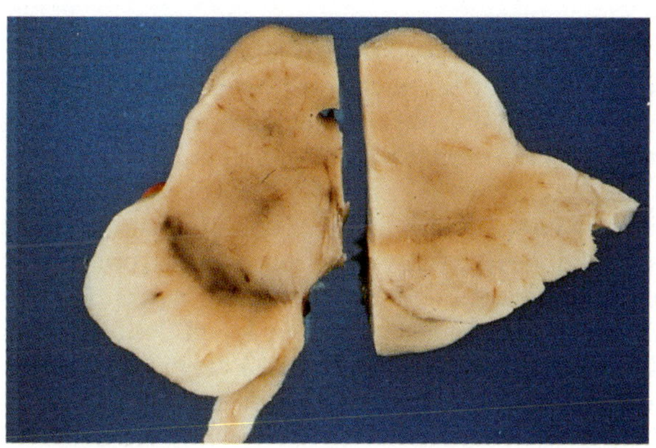

Left: Normal midbrain with heavily pigmented substantia nigra.
Right: Midbrain of a parkinsonian patient showing almost complete loss of pigment from the region of the locus niger.

Lewy bodies: the histological feature of Parkinson's disease

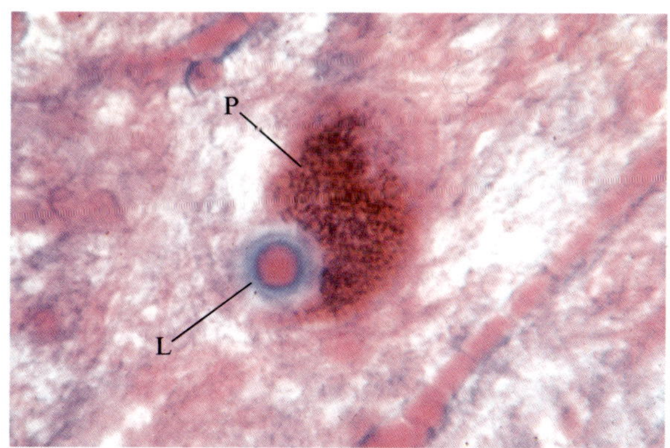

P = Pigment in a neuron
L = Lewy body

Lewy bodies are found in certain cerebral nuclei such as the locus coeruleus, pons, basal nucleus and other areas of the brainstem.

A Rare Virus Infection of the Brain, Leading to Dementia

Creutzfeldt-Jakob disease is a brain disease associated with dementia and various neurological disturbances. It usually leads to the death of the patient in a matter of months. The principal neurological symptom is myoclonic muscle twitches. Typical EEG changes are sometimes noted.

The histological changes in Creutzfeldt-Jakob disease are not very striking. They comprise vesicle-like swellings of the pre- and postsynaptic neuronal processes and a strong astrocyte reaction throughout the grey matter. The cerebral cortex is very frequently affected, and so are sometimes the basal ganglia and cerebellum.

It is important to keep this slow virus disease in mind, since occasionally the highly infectious and resistant virus is transmitted iatrogenically from person to person by tissue transplants and electrodes. Clearly therefore persons with neurological disease should not be accepted as organ or blood donors, especially as Creutzfeldt-Jakob disease is often very difficult to diagnose from the clinical findings. In reviewing the different forms of dementia, it is important to note that some cases of Creutzfeldt-Jakob disease exhibit amyloid-containing plaques similar to those seen in Alzheimer's disease.

Creutzfeldt-Jakob disease is a transmissible virus infection of the brain leading to dementia. It is thought to be caused by an atypical virus. It is calculated that one per million of the population dies of Creutzfeldt-Jakob disease annually.

The histology of Creutzfeldt-Jakob disease

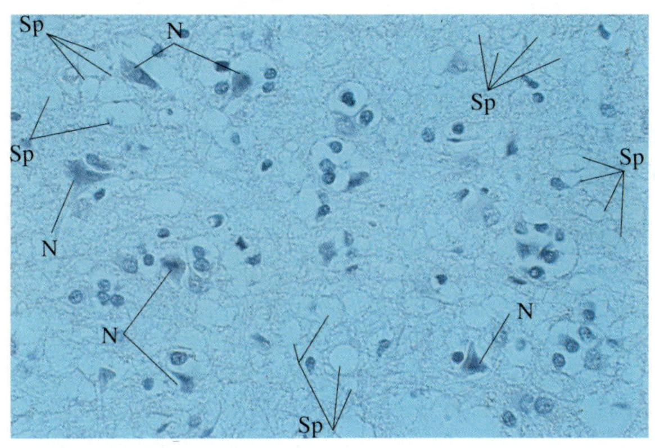

N = Neuron
Sp = Spongiform microcyst

The principal histological feature of Creutzfeldt-Jakob disease is a microcystic degeneration of the neuropil.

The electron microscopic picture of Creutzfeldt-Jakob disease

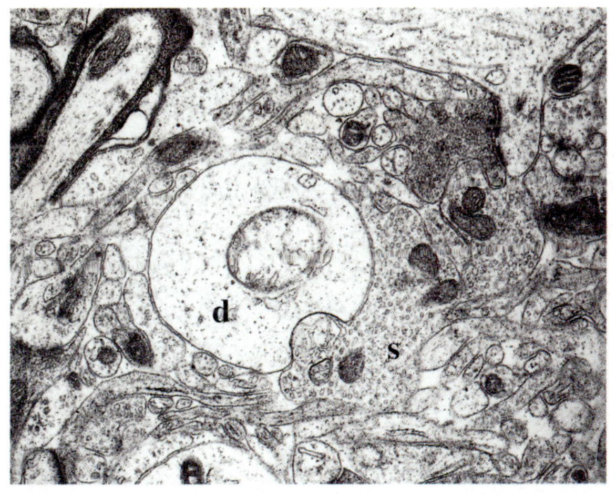

d = Dilated dendrite
s = Presynaptic process showing numerous synaptic vesicles

The electron microscope reveals greatly dilated dendrites; these are the microcytes seen under the light microscope.

Pick's Disease and Brain Disease Associated with Argyrophilic Bodies, Two Uncommon Diseases Leading to Dementia

Arnold Pick, who first described *Pick's disease,* called it circumscribed brain atrophy. Usually the frontal and temporal lobes are affected and the atrophic areas stand out sharply against unaffected cerebral cortex. The affected areas show characteristic changes: intracytoplasmic argyrophilic bodies (Pick bodies) and grossly swollen neurons. It is a rare disease, only about 1 case occurring every 2 years per million of the population. Typically, Pick's disease occurs between the age of 55 and 65 years.

Pick's disease cannot be distinguished clinically from Alzheimer's disease. It proves fatal within a few years (approximately 3–5 years). Although Pick's bodies have an ultrastructure different from that of Alzheimer's neurofibrillary change, they give very similar immunohistochemical reactions. Some of the grossly swollen neurons also show similar reactions.

Age-related dementia associated with argyrophilic granules (Braak) is a disease affecting very old people. About 1 in 20 demented patients is suffering from this disease. As far as is known (the disease was first described in 1987!), this form of dementia does not differ clinically from Alzheimer's disease. The brains of patients with this disease contain granules with a diameter of 2–5 μm, which stain like Alzheimer neurofibrils. It is interesting to note, however, that their ultrastructure differs from that of Alzheimer neurofibrils. It is possible that this disease is a particular manifestation of Alzheimer's disease.

Some cases of senile and presenile dementia are due to less common diseases, such as Pick's disease and brain disease associated with argyrophilic granules. Their relation to Alzheimer's disease has yet to be elucidated.

Diagram showing the distribution of local cerebrocortical atrophy

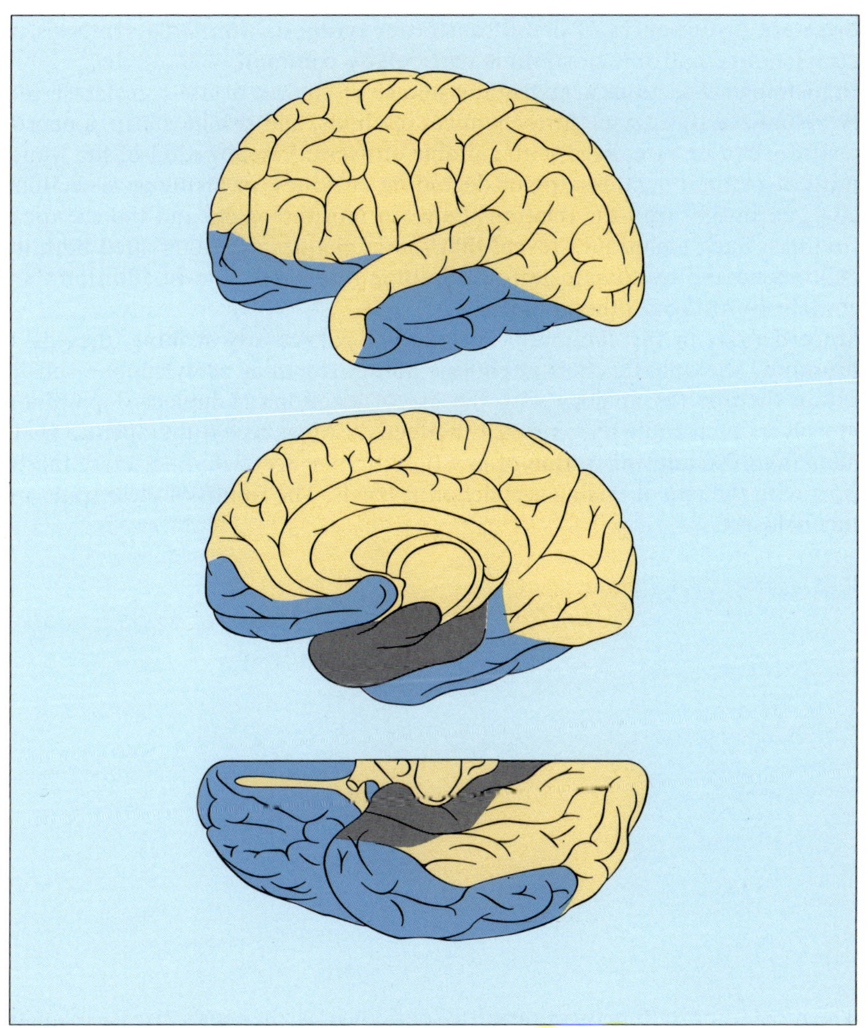

Pick's disease is characterized by atrophy of strictly circumscribed areas of the frontal and/or temporal lobes.

The Neurochemistry of Alzheimer's Disease

In addition to the morphological changes in Alzheimer's disease already described, chemical abnormalities are observed, and the most important of these are disturbances of neurotransmitter synthesis. Impaired synthesis of acetylcholine and somatostatin is particularly common.

In histological sections acetylcholinesterase or choline acetyl-transferase can be visualized by enzyme histochemical methods, and somatostatin, a neuropeptide, can be visualized with suitable antisera. Visualization of the transmitters, or their synthesizing or degrading enzymes, in histological sections gives an insight into the relations between morphological and the chemical findings. Such techniques reveal that senile plaques are innervated both by cholinergic and by somatostatin-containing fibres, but that in addition they contain fibres from other systems.

Since deficits in the cholinergic system are particularly striking, they have prompted therapeutic trials of choline administered as acetylcholine substitution therapy (by analogy with the use of levodopa to replace dopamine). However, such trials have proved ineffective. Most recent therapeutic trials have involved administration of prostigmine-like acetylcholinesterase inhibitors with the aim of raising acetylcholine levels. The results of these trials are inconclusive.

The most important neurotransmitter deficits in Alzheimer's disease relate to acetylcholine and somatostatin. Observation of deficits of these neurotransmitters has prompted various attempts at substitution therapy.

Visualization of the acetylcholinesterase reaction in plaques

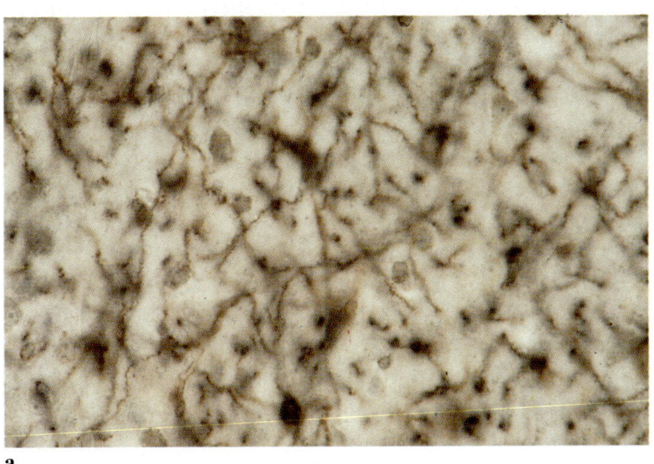

a

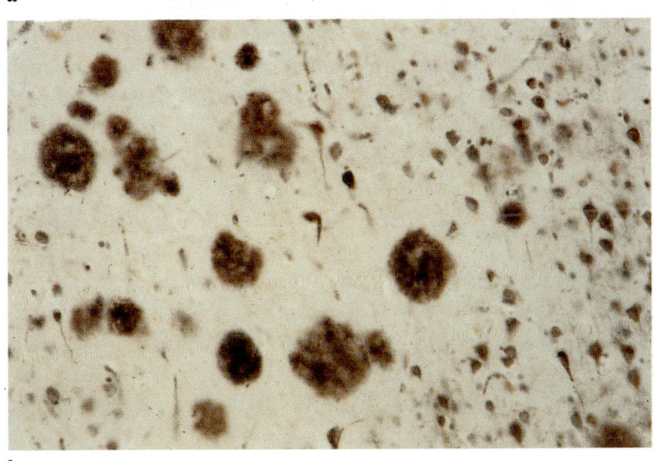

b

Comparison of acetylcholinesterase activity visualized by enzyme histochemical methods in normal cerebral cortex (**a**) and in Alzheimer's disease (**b**) indicates that the plaques exhibit marked acetylcholinesterase activity, Furthermore, the network of cholinergic nerve fibres seen in the normal brain disappears.

The Aetiology of Alzheimer's Disease

The cause of Alzheimer's disease is unknown. The probability of developing the disease increases with age. In recent years genetic studies of some families have shown that Alzheimer's disease conforms to an autosomal-dominant pattern of inheritance. The question of whether a precentage of the senile, supposedly sporadic, manifestations of Alzheimer's disease in old age are hereditary is very difficult to answer. Some observations point to additional exogenous factors, such as repeated brain trauma or chronic intoxication.

It is well established that a large proportion of professional boxers develop dementia. Interestingly enough, boxers' brains display a massive increase in Alzheimer's neurofibrillary change, but only a few plaques. These changes have been shown to correlate with the number of brain traumas received in boxing bouts (knock-outs).

Statistical studies on Alzheimer patients have revealed that a history of cranial injury or brain damage is more common in Alzheimer patients than in the general population. When their history is taken, patients should therefore always be questioned about such incidents.

With regard to chronic intoxication as a cause of Alzheimer's disease, the finger of suspicion has been pointed inter alia at aluminium. The evidence for the possible implication of aluminium is twofold:

(1) In laboratory animals and tissue cultures aluminium salts induce marked cytoskeletal changes in neurons, these changes resembling Alzheimer neurofibrils.

(2) Increased quantities of aluminium have been detected in the brains of patients with Alzheimer's disease, especially in brain regions showing Alzheimer changes.

However, the increased level of aluminium may not play a causal role in Alzheimer's disease. It is conceivable, for example, that the proteins of plaques and tangles might have a particular affinity for aluminium, and thus accumulate it by adsorption. Moreover, it should be borne in mind that aluminium is one of the commonest elements on the earth's surface and therefore occurs in all living tissues.

Genetic factors certainly play a part in the development of Alzheimer's disease. Furthermore, the current thinking is that there might conceivably be a link between Alzheimer's disease and cranial injury, brain damage and intoxication.

Experimentally induced Alzheimer's neurofibrillary change

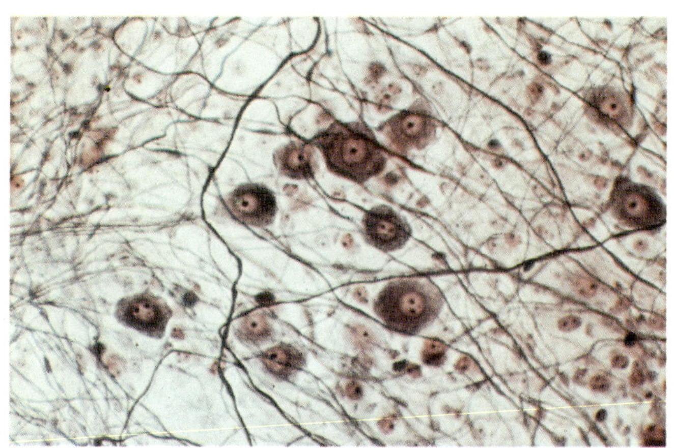

Normal neurons in tissue culture.

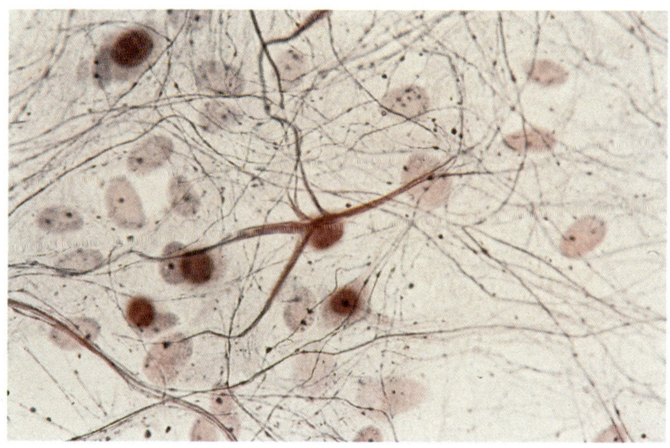

Neurons stained as above. Aluminium added to the culture medium has induced cytoskeletal changes similar to Alzheimer fibrils [after D. Langui].

Early Diagnosis of Dementing Disorders of Old Age

B. Fischer, S. Lehrl, H. Woelk, U. Fischer

Age Can Be Defined according to Different Criteria

Clinical diagnosis of the transition from normal to pathological aging is one of the great challenges facing medical science in our time. What do we mean by age and aging?

In addition to *chronological age,* which simply refers to the number of years a person has lived, there is the concept of *functional age.* This can be further divided into biological (or physiological), psychological and social age.

Biological age is an expression of overall physical/physiological function, while *psychological age* reflects the level of adjustment to one's environment, and *social age* one's age as a function of social situation or role. For example, a 40-year-old football player is considered very old, a 40-year-old President very young.

A useful rule for the *'prognosis of aging'* is: The better a person has coped with the social relationships and social problems encountered in the previous phase of life, the greater are his chances of success in the subsequent phase.

Subjective age – how old a person feels – is of decisive importance for future life prospects. Individuals who have an optimistic view of the future can expect to live an average of 10 years longer than those who do not.

Depending on the standpoint of the observer, age can be divided into:

- chronological age (years lived),
- functional age:
  - biological age (a person's general physiological state),
  - psychological age (psychological adaptability),
  - social age (functioning in social context),
- subjective age (how old a person feels; inner vitality).

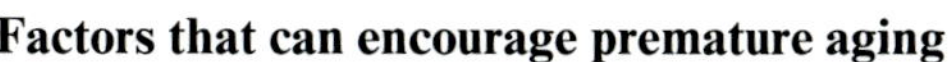

Factors that can encourage premature aging

Negative childhood memories
Early death of parents, emotional precocity
Happiest time of life before the age of 30
Period of greatest achievement by the age of 30–40
Low-status occupation, work perceived as unsuitable
Undemanding job, failure to achieve life goals
Work in large rooms, under stress
Dissatisfaction with job, tendency to have passive interests or none at all
Unfavourable economic situation, life marked by a negative preoccupation with the past, the present appears burdensome and joyless
Passive attitude to life, preoccupation with physical complaints
Inflexible in coping with frustrations, susceptibility to 'functional' disturbances
Preference for solitude or exclusive company of spouse
Narrow interests
Irregular sleep, marked susceptibility to diseases

Minimal abilities that must be preserved in order to reduce the risk of death

The ability to walk 2 km (1.4 miles)
The ability to lift about 5 kg (11 lbs)
The ability to walk up 10 steps without pausing for breath
The ability to crawl, crouch and kneel
A normal intelligence quotient
Mental flexibility

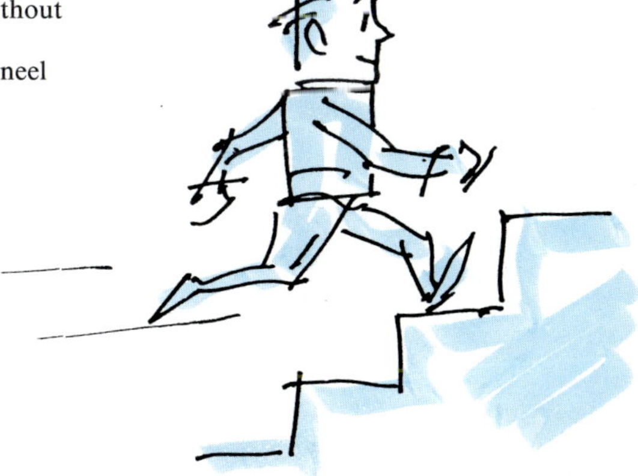

Involutional Physiological Changes Affecting Brain Function

Physiological aging is primarily the result of aging of the nerve cells of the brain and sensory organs. Only in very advanced old age is there a reduction in the number of neurons (in healthy individuals). Before this the neurons will show at most some degree of atrophy. It has been postulated that this occurs when nerve cells are underused ('understimulated'). The number of synapses likewise increases or decreases depending on their use. Experiments have shown that animals in old people's homes and similar environments have markedly fewer synapses than animals kept in stimulating environments. Even physical training on an exercise bicycle at 25–50 W increases mental agility.

The following changes in motor function are seen in the elderly:

- decline of capacity of perform integrated movements;
- overall motor retardation;
- slowing of individual movements;
- slowing of movement initiation;
- decreased need to move the trunk;
- need to move the head and hands remains normal;
- the 'physiological' changes in motor function can have a negative effect on cerebral blood flow and cerebral metabolism;
- physiologically, psychologically and socially there is a decline in regulatory range and adaptability.

A combination of daily mental (10 min) and physical (25–50 W) exercises is essential for the preservation of neurons and synapses in old age.

One hour of mental exercise preserves nerve cells and mental function in old age

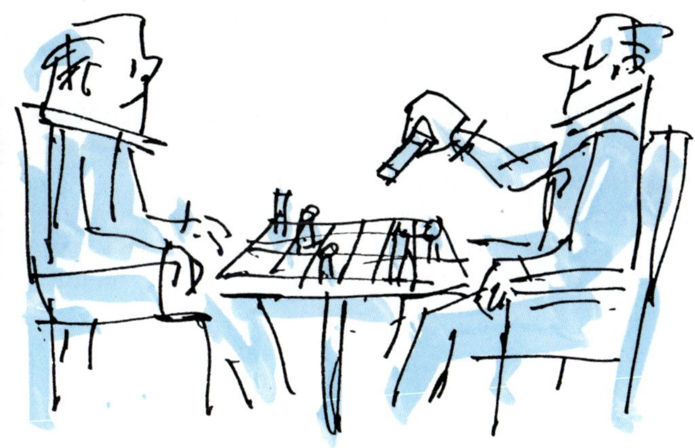

A moderate keep-fit programme helps to maintain not only physical but mental agility

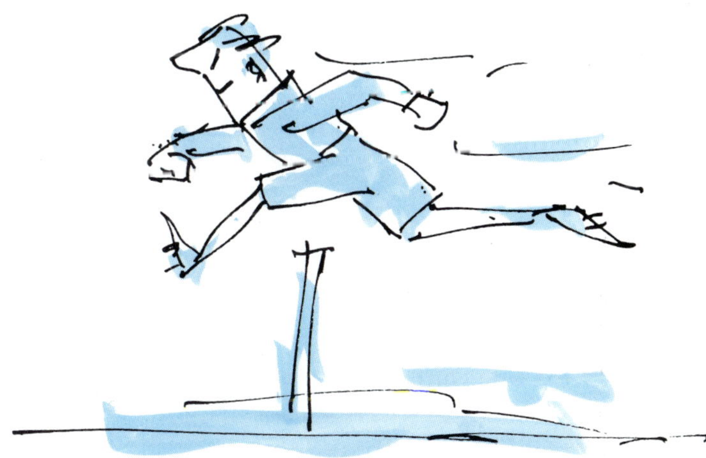

The Meaning of Senile Dementia

Much confusion has been engendered by inconsistent use of the term (senile) dementia to denote intellectual deterioration in old age, and many terms have been and are still used as synonyms. These include: chronic brain failure, psycho-organic syndrome, organic brain syndrome, Alzheimer's disease, organic psychosis, diffuse cerebrovascular disease and diffuse cerebral atrophy.

Today the term senile dementia is often used to mean intellectual impairment of organic origin which is generally permanent and progressive, although it should not be linked to the idea of irreversibility.

Organic brain syndrome would probably be a more comprehensive term, particularly since it does not appear to automatically exclude personality loss and emotional deterioration. However, the term senile dementia is retained here for the sake of standardization.

To be consistent with current usage the term senile dementia is used in this article, reserving the expression Alzheimer's disease for the early form of dementia (presenile dementia).

The term senile dementia covers a multitude of different concepts and entities

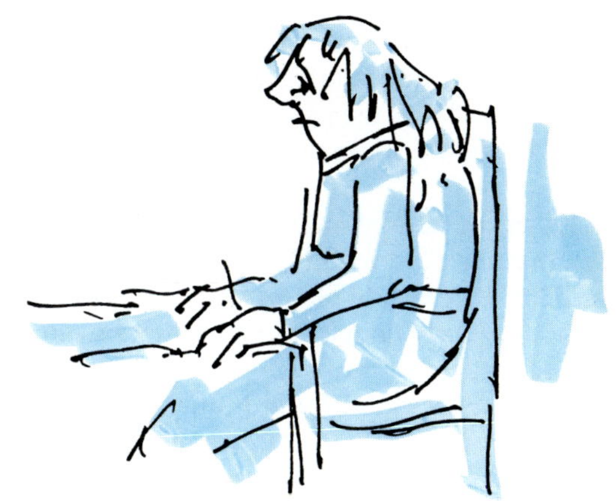

Organic brain syndrome and its principal subtypes (including synonymous expressions)

Organic brain syndrome
(= psycho-organic syndrome)
(= brain failure)

Acute organic brain syndrome
(= reversible organic psychosis)
(= symptomatic psychosis)

Chronic organic brain syndrome or senile dementia
(= irreversible organic psychosis)

Patients with chronic organic brain syndrome may exhibit features of both subtypes.

Prevalence in Incidence of Senile Dementia

In 2030 about 25% of the population in Europe and 20% in the USA will be over 65 years of age.
The frequency (prevalence) of senile dementia is estimated to be 5% in those over the age of 65 and 20% in those over 80.
Epidemiological studies carried out in the Federal Republic of Germany in 1988 found that the prevalence of severe dementia among people over the age of 65 was 4.9% (465,000 cases) and that of mild dementia 8.7% (826,000 cases).
The mean annual rate for newly diagnosed cases (incidence) is over 1%, increasing exponentially with age, while the proportion of severe dements among residents of old people's homes (at present about 50%) is greater than among elderly people living in their own homes. However, when considering these figures it must be borne in mind that 86% of patients with senile dementia are cared for at home.
The average *duration of illness* is 5–10 years, with life expectancy decreasing the earlier the onset of the disease and the more marked the deterioration of cognitive funciton.
In the USA senile dementia or dementia of the Alzheimer type is listed in the mortality statistics as the 4th–5th commonest cause of death.

Senile dementia is a common illness of old age, affecting 5% of those over the age of 65 and 20% of those over 80.

Forms of senile dementia

The following frequency distribution for the various forms of dementia is generally accepted:

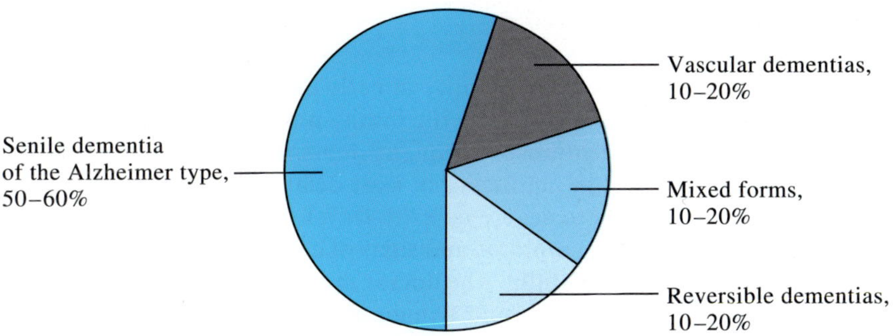

The risk of developing senile dementia increases with age!

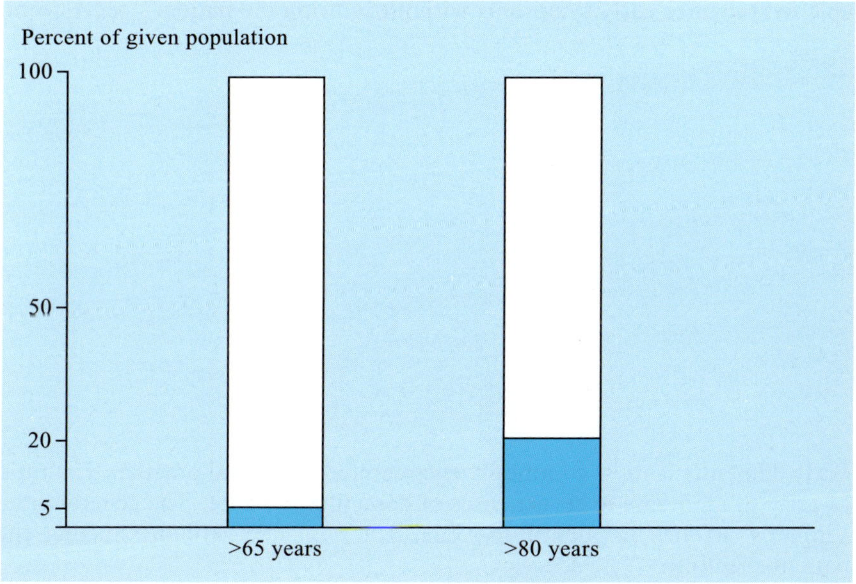

Percent of given population

100

50

20

5

>65 years

>80 years

Memory Impairment Must Always Be Taken Seriously as a Sign of Possible Dementia

Symptoms such as:
- poor concentration,
- increased fatigability,
- difficulty in recalling names and recent events,
- diminished vitality,
- mental rigidity,
- mood swings

should alert the doctor to the possibility of early dementia. In practice, 80% of early cases remain undiagnosed by the family physician (iceberg phenomenon). The early identification of incipient dementia is important since it offers a realistic prospect of halting, or at least delaying, its progression. The ratio of mild to moderate to severe cases is 14:7:1, but general practitioners must be familiar with the symptoms and signs of early dementia if they are to recognize and treat it successfully. The doctor must be capable of distinguishing between incipient dementia and benign age-associated memory impairment.

Diagnosis is often made difficult by the fact that the patient is unable to accept the symptoms and so tries to conceal them. The doctor must thus be able to recognize early symptoms without injuring the patient's self-esteem.

Early dementia is most commonly encountered in general practice. The ratio of early to moderate to severe cases of dementia is 14:7:1. The general practitioner's art lies in identifying incipient dementia without hurting the patient's feelings.

The iceberg phenomenon of early senile dementia

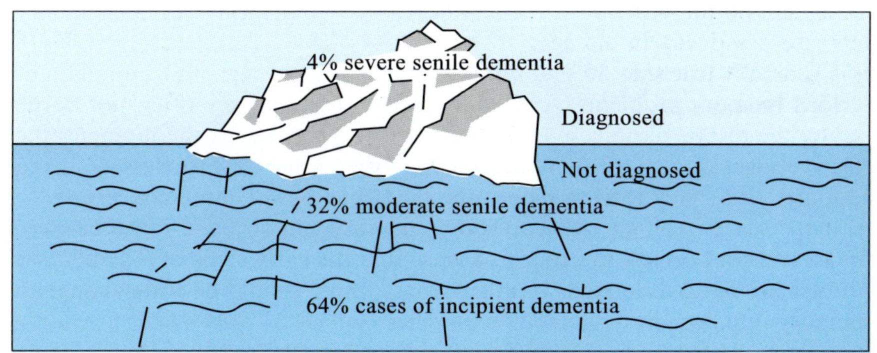

Moderate degrees of senile dementia and early stages of dementing brain disease are generally not recognized and therefore treated too late.

Early symptoms of senile dementia are often disguised by the fact that the patient systematically refuses to acknowledge their existence

I'm happy
because I can still
remember everything

... and I'm happy
because I can
forget everything

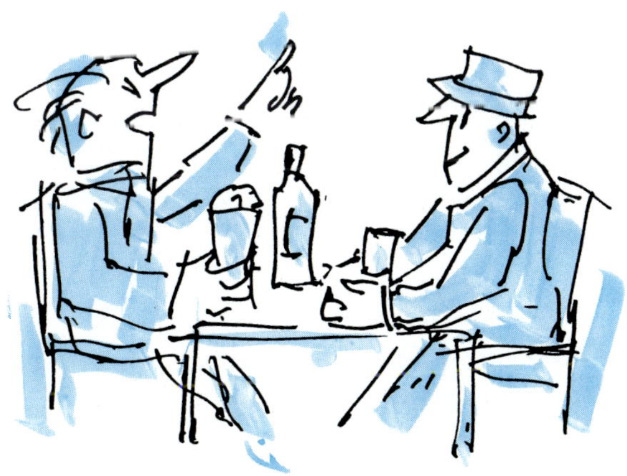

The Need for Caution in Diagnosing Benign Age-Associated Memory Impairment

Benign age-associated memory impairment is characterized principally by mild forgetfulness. There is no loss of mental function relevant to everyday living and no impairment of cortical functions. Complaints of poor memory increase drastically in old age.

It is generally true that 50% of normal people over the age of 60 complain of serious memory problems. And while their complaints are often not borne out by the results of objective memory tests – ignoring, for the moment, the relative insensitivity of many such tests – they must nevertheless be taken seriously since they tend to determine the behaviour of those concerned.

A diagnosis of benign age-associated memory impairment must be kept under constant review in order to ensure that the early signs of a dementing process are not overlooked. In other words, there should be little change in memory impairment over months or years.

Benign age-associated memory impairment	Method of diagnosis	
	clinical	psychometric
Memory impairment	+	+
Disorientation	0	0
Inappropriate conversational remarks	0	0
Impaired sense of well-being	++	++
Personality deterioration	0	0
Difficulty with everyday tasks	0	0

The diagnosis of benign age-associated memory impairment should be reviewed at 4- to 6-month intervals to minimize the risk of missing the onset of personality deterioration dementia.

The doctor's response to memory impairment is often ridicule rather than careful diagnosis

'It's awful how forgetful my husband has become', the wife complains to the consultant. 'I can talk on and on to him for hours on end but when I've finished, he doesn't remember a word I've said'.
'That, madam', says the consultant, smiling, 'is not memory loss, it's a blessing!'

Patterns of memory impairment in old age

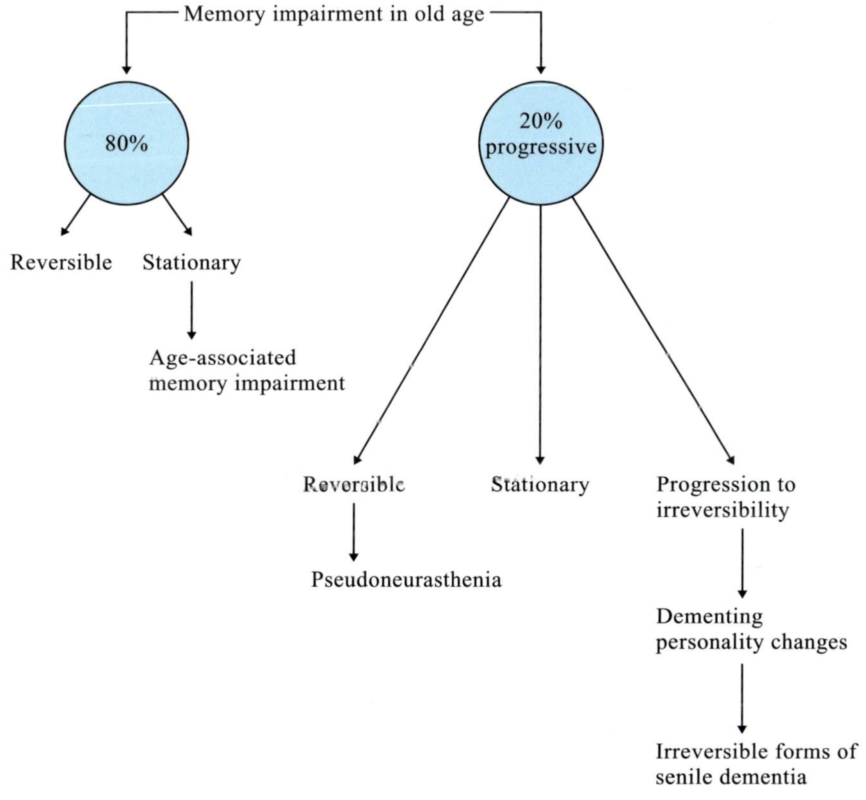

Impaired Information Processing in Early Senile Dementia

The processing of information by the brain is controlled chiefly by the centres for fluid and crystallized intelligence.

Fluid intelligence is defined by several authors as the ability to perceive and comprehend complex relationships in new situations. This includes tasks requiring inductive thought and associative abilities.

Fluid intelligence is a combination of two factors:

(1) information processing speed (15 bits/s), and

(2) immediate retention (short-term memory; retention time 5.4 s).

Multiplication of the two factors yields the short-term storage capacity, the decisive variable for coping with everday life.

Disturbances occurring in the early phases of dementia involve mainly fluid intelligence, which is associated with short-term memory. Deterioration of long-term and preconscious memory, which are closely linked with *crystallized intelligence,* is seen only in advanced senile dementia.

By analogy with information processing we can distinguish between two forms of intelligence:

fluid intelligence, which is closely linked with short-term memory, and crystallized intelligence, which depends on the memory's long-term storage capacity. Fluid intelligence is the decisive factor for the performance of everyday tasks.

Information processing model (psychostructural model)

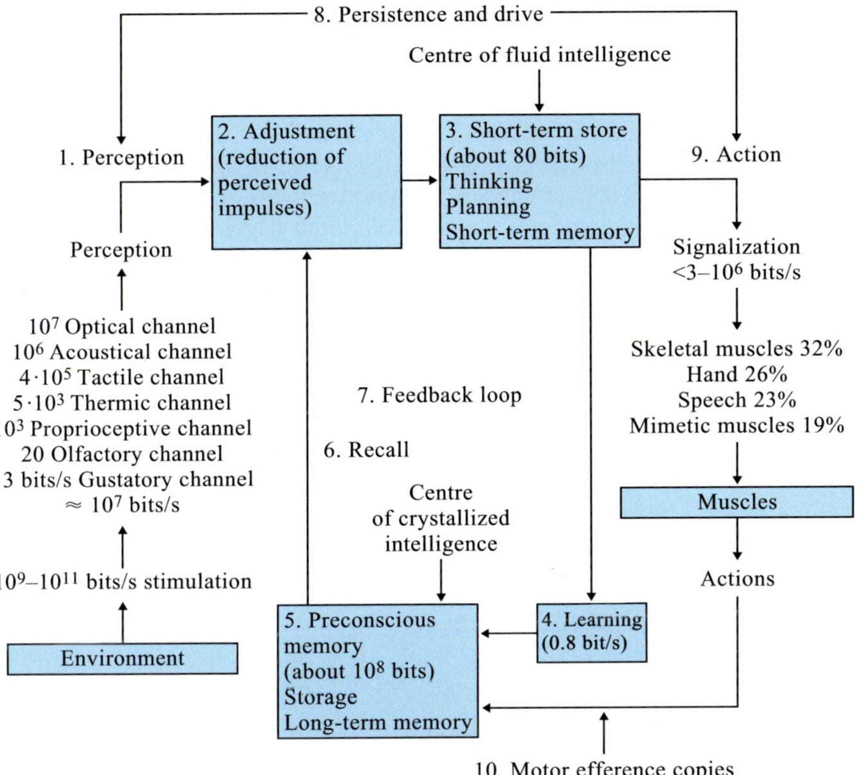

Environmental stimuli are perceived at a rate of 10^9–10^{11} bits/s, while the sensory organs are capable of transmitting at 10^7 bits/s. This deluge of stimuli is reduced to 15 bits/s by adjustment and fed into the short-term memory (processing speed × immediate retention), which has a capacity of about 80 bis. Of these, 0.8 bits/s are stored in the preconscious memory (the seat of crystallized intelligence), which has a capacity of about 10^8 bits. From here information can be retrieved and fed back into the cycle for 'readjustment' and processing by the short-term memory.

Fluid and Crystallized Intelligence Are Altered in the Early Stages of Senile Dementia

The key determinants of mental capacity in both youth and old age are:
(1) innate intellectual aptitude,
(2) the extent of environmental demands and memory use,
(3) an intact sensory system (sight, hearing, smell, touch, taste),
(4) permanent question grid,
(5) mental attitude to problems (intentionality) and basic dimension of self-awareness (reflexivity).

As far as the memory's short-term storage capacity (= fluid intelligence) is concerned, intellectual capability has reached its peak by the 16th year of life. Beyond this age it begins to show a gradual decline, not least as a result of inadequate use. This tendency can be accelerated by biological stresses (in particular heart and lung diseases), as well as psychological and negative social factors. Short-term storage capacity is affected particularly seriously in the early stages of dementia.

The long-term storage capacity of the brain (crystallized intelligence) encompasses the following:
- vocabulary (understanding of language, general knowledge, empirical knowledge),
- judgement,
- the ability to conceptualize, to think logically and in abstract terms, to reason and draw conclusions and to solve problems (strategies, metastrategies),
- the ability to grasp connections between ideas,
- the critical faculty, sense of priorities, capacity for self-reflection,
- insight into physical and mental changes (e.g. due to disease).

In early forms of dementing brain disease, crystallized intelligence and long-term memory remain unaffected longer than fluid intelligence and short-term memory.

Normal and pathological decline in intellectual function in relation to age

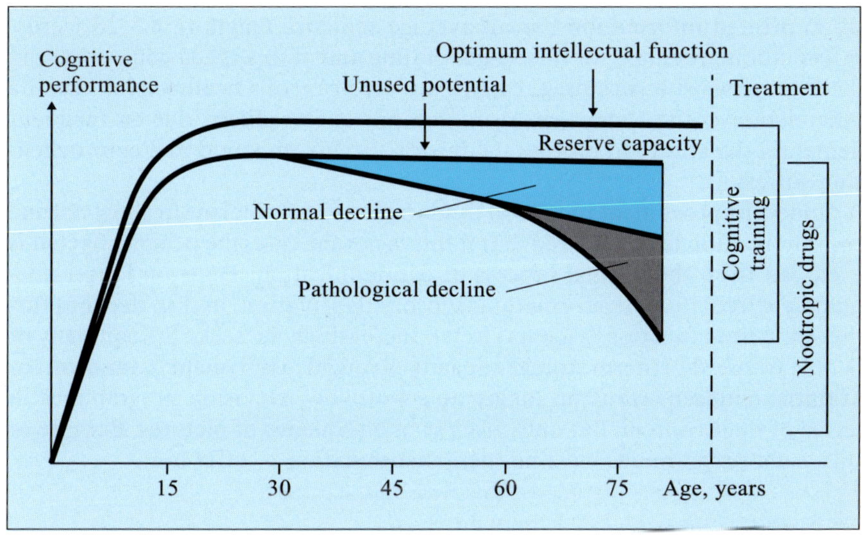

Normal, 'age-related' decline in intellectual function can be compensated for by mental (cognitive) training but a pathological decline must be tackled by a combined approach. This consists of general management of any underlying disorders (e.g. heart failure, thyreotoxicosis, blood flow disorders), cognitive training and treatment with drugs capable of stimulating cerebral activity, such as Hydergine.

Impairment of Routine Mental (Cognitive) Abilities in Early Dementia

Maintenance of the short-term storage capacity of the brain is essential since impairment reduces the ability to cope with routine tasks such as orientation in traffic or shopping without a shopping list. Important sources of new information – and hence of mental stimulation – are direct communication between marriage partners, information heard on the radio or television and information read in newspapers and magazines.

In general, oral information is presented in the form of sentences lasting about 5 s (maximum 8 s) at the normal speaking rate of about 2.5 words/s, while printed information has an average sentence length of 12–28 words. Information presented for this length of time and at this speed will not exceed the average short-term storage capacity of the brain of a healthy adult. On the other hand, if the short-term storage capacity is reduced due to incipient dementia the ability to process the information is impaired and comprehension suffers.

A modest improvement in mental function is often sufficient to allow normal communication to be restored, but if this is not the case, the person affected is excluded from the normal process of communication. He is no longer adequately stimulated by information (sensory deprivation) and so declines further in mental function (vicious circle). Increasingly he seeks the company of people whose short-term storage capacity is roughly equivalent to his own, for example children. He is no longer able to follow television programmes in terms of their content, but only visually as a sequence of pictures. Because of this, such programmes have no mental stimulation to offer him.

Normal communication is impossible if the brain's short-term information storage capacity is impaired.

The defective communication grid for information processing in early senile dementia

The defective communication grid at the limit of normal

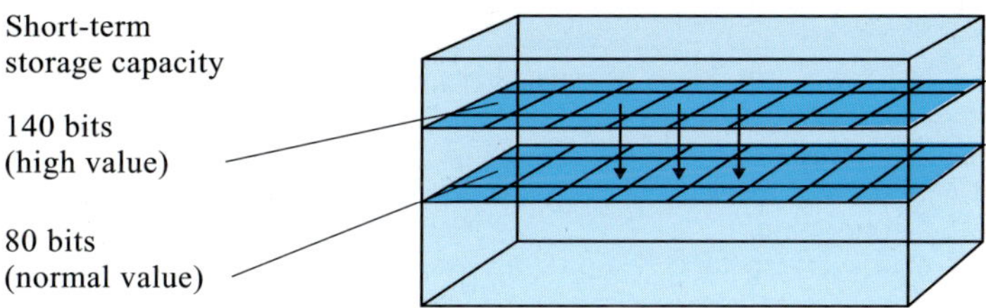

As long as it does not fall below the normal value, a reduction in the short-term storage capacity of the brain leads to feelings of distress. The patient notices that his intellectual powers have deteriorated. He suffers from short-term memory difficulties, poor concentration and emotional lability. He is still quite able to follow normal communication but generally tires more easily.

The failing communication grid

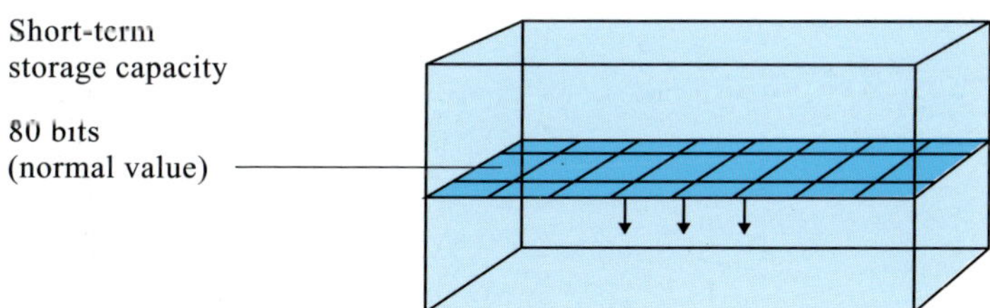

A fall in the short-term storage capacity from a normal initial level means to drop through the communication grid. The patient can no longer follow normal communication.

Clinical Diagnosis of Early Dementia

The early stages of dementing processes are characterized above all by a decline in cognitive processing abilities, usually accompanied by an impaired sense of well-being and changes in personality structure.
Early dementia can be identified on the basis of the following clinical and psychometric features:

	Clinical	Psychometric
Intellectual deterioration	+	+
Impaired sense of well-being	++	++
Personality deterioration	0/+	0/+
Difficulties with everyday tasks	0/+	0/+

Two of the criteria are of decisive importance for the diagnosis of early dementia:
(1) increasing decline in mental function,
(2) personality changes (although this is not closely correlated with the decline in cognitive function).

Deterioration of cognitive processing abilities and an impaired sense of well-being are typical of early dementia. This process is often associated with personality changes.

Symptoms of impaired intellectual processing, sense of well-being and personality structure in early dementia

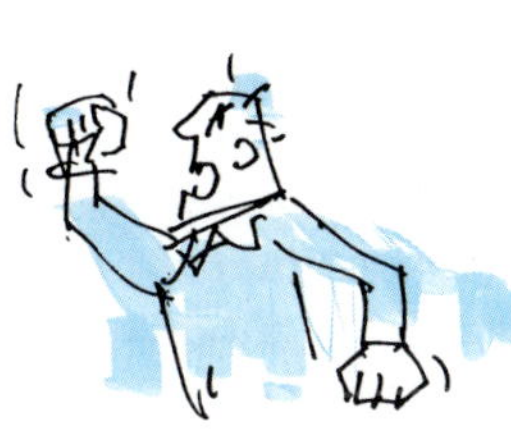

Impairment of cognitive processing

Attention ↓
Comprehension, perception ↓
Thinking, planning ↓
Learning, memory, remembering ↓
Communication with partner (e.g. conversation) ↓
Communication with environment (e.g. stereoscopic vision, orientation, time, place, person, situation) ↓
Psychomotor speed ↓

↓

'Staying power' and drive ↓

↓

Higher cognitive processes (e.g. lack of insight) ↓

Impaired sense of well-being

Loss of vitality
Emotional instability
(irritability at cognitive overload, etc.)

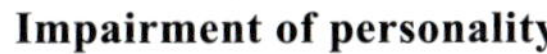

Impairment of personality

Hypertypical:
e.g. caricaturing of character (the miser becomes more miserly, the talker more talkative)
Mental rigidity, indecisiveness

Hypotypical:
Dwindling of personality

Heterotypical:
Restructuring of personality
e.g. loss of learned social inhibitions, bill dodging, sexual misbehaviour

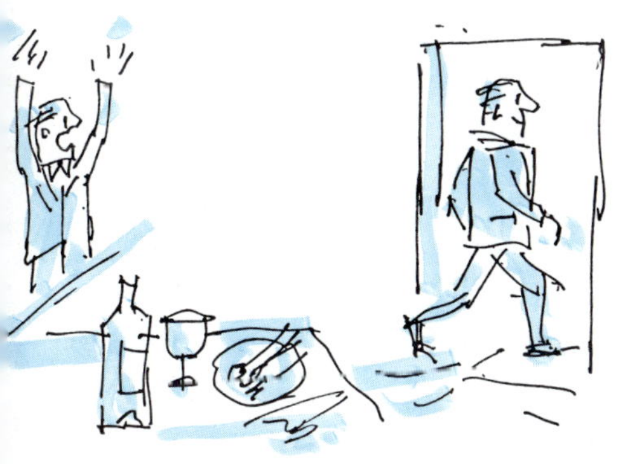

Early Dementia and Impaired Cognitive Processing

Impaired cognitive processing manifests itself as difficulty in the conscious perception of events occurring in one's environment. There is loss of interest, poor concentration, and difficulty in switching attention quickly from one thing to another. Above all there is a loss of the ability to select information and relate new information to what is already known.

Information processing speed and immediate retention are diminished. For example, there is an inability to understand long sentences (whether read or heard), to grasp complex sentence structures, to read quickly or understand rapid speech.

There is a learning deficit (encoding deficit) for all sensory inputs other than pain. This is particularly striking if two tasks have to be accomplished at the same time; when given the second one to solve, the patient immediately forgets the original task.

An information retrieval deficit is shown by an inability to recognize objects, names or people. Nor can newly learnt information be retrieved at a later time, as is often the case in benign senescent forgetfulness.

Communication difficulties arise because information is processed at a much 'shallower' level.

Disorientation in time, space and situation, shallower information processing, learning deficits and impaired short-term memory are the key symptoms of a dementing personality change.

Cardinal symptoms of impaired information processing in the context of dementing personality change

Early symptoms of senile dementia (according to the psychostructural model, see p. 49)
- Perceptual dysfunction
- Impairment of information selection (associative memory; accommodation failure = impairment of information restriction)
- Quantitatively reduced information processing (encoding and retrieval deficits, with impaired orientation with regard to time, space and situation)
- Reduced short-term memory (retrieval deficit = impaired recall)
- Learning deficit (encoding deficit)
- Lack of persistence in performance of tasks
- Loss of vitality (decreased drive and motivation; truncated or inappropriate actions)

Verbal communication problems (spontaneous speech) in early dementia
- Forgetting or abruptly changing topic of conversation
- Loss of ability to repeat a story ('loses thread')
- Inappropriate remarks in rapidly changing conversational situations
- Comprehension difficulties (with sayings, abstract concepts, humour, irony, sarcasm, etc.)
- Problems of communication with environment [impaired orientation with regard to time, place, person and situation (earliest changes)]
- Confabulation (attempt to compensate for impaired verbal communication)
- Loss of vitality (diminished 'staying power', drive and motivation)
- Truncated or inappropriate actions (reacting differently to familiar surroundings, agitation, restless hyperactivity and wandering)
- In familiar surroundings social competence often remains (at least partially) intact for a considerable time

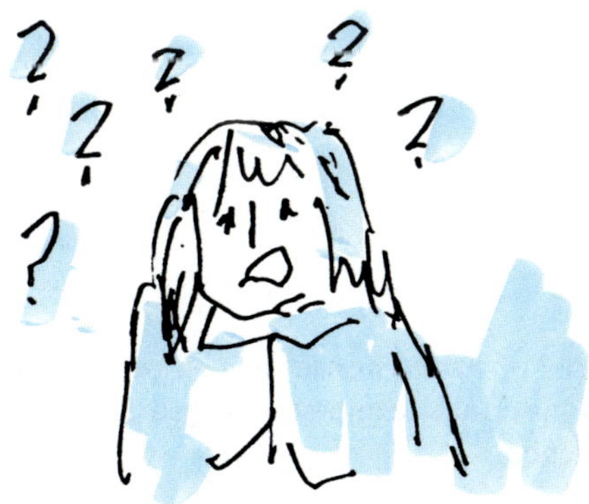

A Lost Sense of Well-Being May Be the First Symptom of Early Dementia

In the early stages of dementia the most conspicuous features of impaired well-being are diminution of vitality and a decline in mental and physical competence. For example, more and more time is needed for routine tasks; the patient is usually aware of this, tries to fight against it, and finds that he can do nothing about the defective information processing. Old behaviours are activated, while new ones cannot be learnt. The patient is easily fatigued by everyday tasks but is unable to sleep.

There is a crumbling of self-esteem, usually associated with a sense of distress initially. The patient is keenly aware of the progressive nature of his deficits and tries to 'react', but the results in general asthenia or loss of emotional equilibrium, with increased self-preoccupation. Irritability (dysphoria) and mood swings or emotional incontinence become increasingly common.

An impaired sense of well-being in early dementia is marked by disturbed emotional responses as well as by a loss of vitality and functional competence.

Symptoms of impaired mental well-being in senile dementia

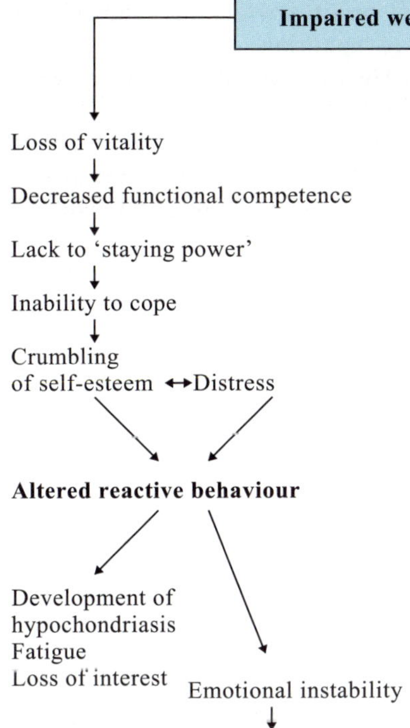

Non-specific and pseudovegetative disorders
Dull headache
('like a tight band around the head')
Tinnitus
Hypersensitivity to sound
Yawning attacks
Increased sweating
Dry mouth on waking
Sleep disturbances
(particularly when dominant cerebral hemisphere is more affected)
Interrupted sleep
Early waking, no feeling of having slept
No memory of dreams
(diminished REM phases)
Fall asleep during the day

General unpleasant sensations
Hypaesthesia
Hypalgesia
Paraesthesia (without organic cause)
Dysuria (without organic cause)

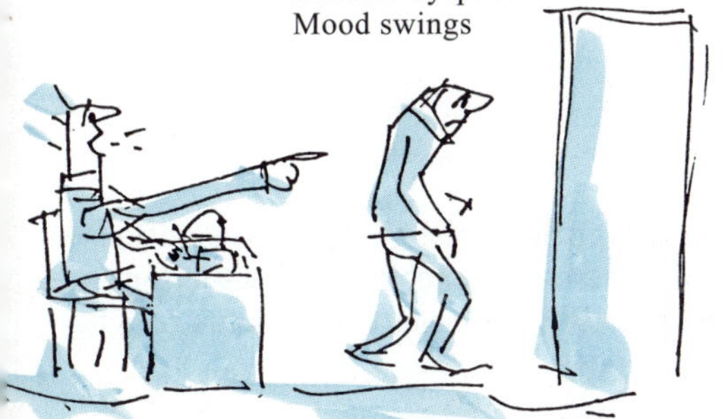

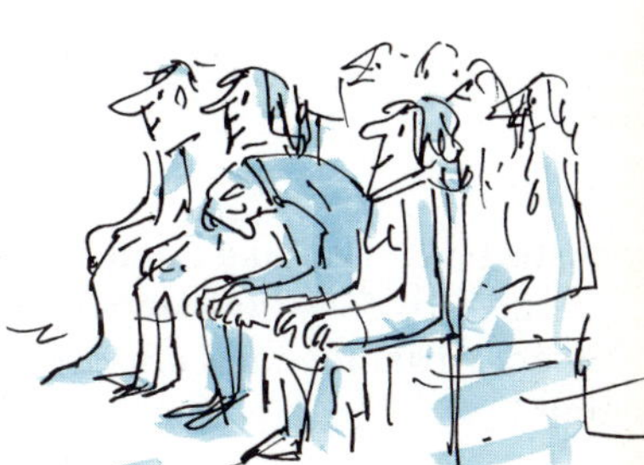

Disturbance of Emotional Equilibrium – A Further Sign of Personality Deterioration

Against a background of diminishing self-esteem, the patient with dementing personality disintegration begins to fear that he may have contracted cancer or some other chronic illness (hypochondriasis). He also experiences increasingly severe fluctuations in mood (emotional lability), which may range from self-centred concern to extreme irritability (dysphoria).

The patient is tired, apathetic and passive. He sits around without interest, incapable of doing anything on his own initiative.

Sometimes the picture is dominated by the patient's extreme concern about his own state of health, any attempt by others to allay or discuss these anxieties being met by hurt or angry reactions. Otherwise he is sullen and yields to fatalistic resignation.

In some cases the patient is aware of his negative behaviour towards the outside world, but is incapable of doing anything effective to counteract it.

Disturbed emotional equilibrium in dementing personality disintegration is characterized by unfounded fear of illness and increasing fluctuations in mood. Irritability and affective hypersensitivity alternate with sullen resignation.

Altered reactive behaviour in early dementia and the inability to develop adequate 'counteractive' strategies

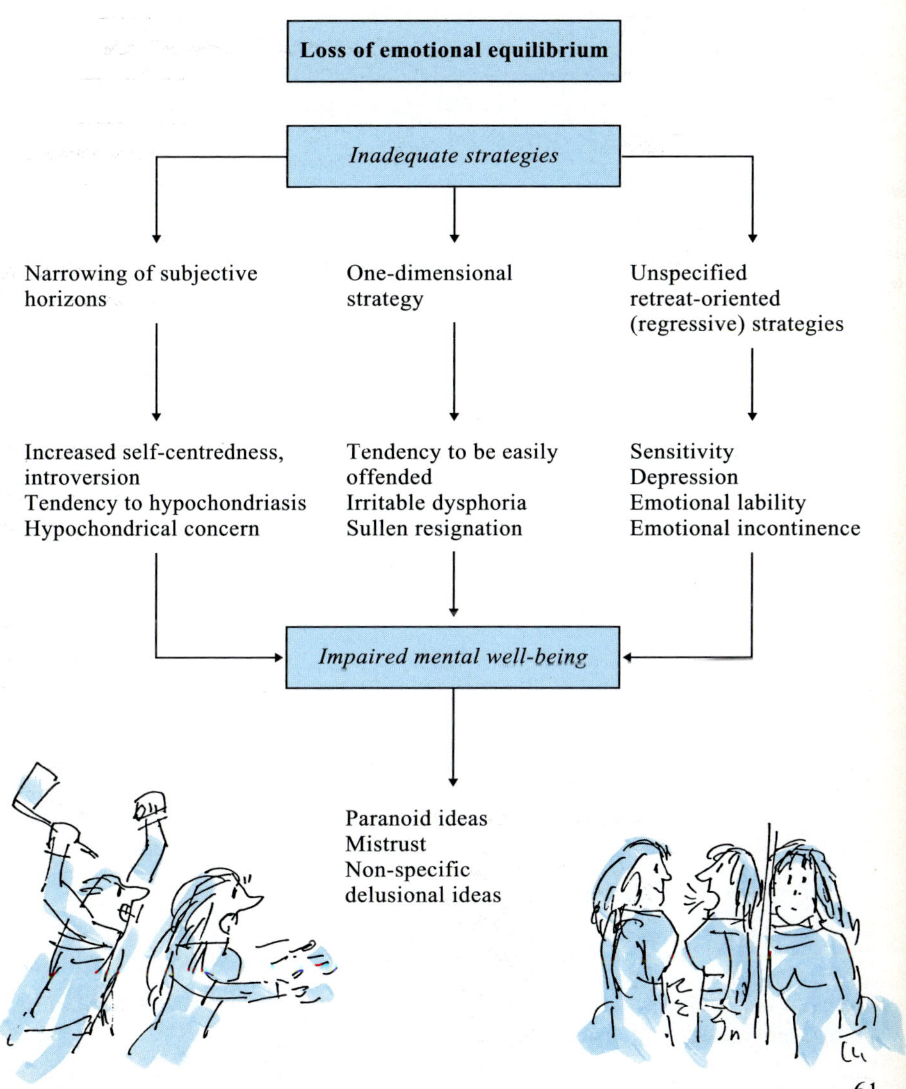

Incidence of Depression in Early Dementia

Endogenous depression is no more common in patients with genuine dementing processes than in normal subjects of comparable age, but an impaired feeling of well-being with mood depression is present in 60% of early cases, 40% of moderately advanced cases and 10% of severe cases.
It is important to distinguish true depression from these emotional reactions, although a number of symptoms overlap. Nevertheless, it was found in a 7-year follow-up study that patients with these features who had early dementia never developed classic depression.

Cases of endogenous depression are no commoner in early dementia than in comparable groups of similar age.

Differential diagnosis between early dementia with mood depression and true depression

Early dementia	Depression
Generally insidious, with indeterminate onset	Rapid, recognizable onset, but no futher progression after short time (follow-up examination)
Onset sometimes sudden in multi-infarct dementia	Previous history of mild depressive and/or manic phases; subsequent hypomanic fluctuations
No delusions	Frequent delusions (e.g. of impoverishment, ill health)
Mood and behaviour fluctuate	Mood consistently depressive
Symptoms persistent	Symptoms often of short duration
Most answers approximately correct	'Dont't know' answers are typical
Patient seeks to conceal deficits	Patient openly displays deficits
Cooperation during examination usually good	Cooperation during examination generally poor
Diurnal fluctuations rare	Diurnal fluctuations common
Refreshed after short sleep	Not refreshed after short sleep
Cognitive impairment relatively constant throughout day	Wide fluctuations in cognitive impairment throughout day
Orientation impaired (time orientation may be affected particularly early)	Orientation normal
Inappropriate conversational remarks, frequently forgets topic of conversation	Appropriate remarks, topic of conversation not forgotten
Difficulties in coping with everyday living tasks	No difficulties in coping with everyday living tasks
Symptoms respond to multidimensional therapy (general management, cerebral stimulation, antidementia drugs, e.g. Hydergine)	Symptoms respond to antidepressants

Senile Dementia Is Usually Accompanied by Personality Changes

The first signs of personality change are often mental rigidity and indecisiveness.

Mental rigidity is a central feature of the incipient personality change. The dwindling of the personality promotes the emergence of certain character traits in exaggerated form, for example, self-centred isolation, obstinacy, insistence on the correctness of one's own opinions, pedantry, fear of innovation.

Often this mental rigidity is accompanied by *indecisiveness,* usually reflecting a profound loss of self-confidence. As the pathological process advances, and knowledge, skills and strategies are no longer able to meet the needs of reality (impairment of cognitive abilities), routine tasks can no longer be performed.

– Indecisiveness
↓
– Inability to perform routine tasks
↓
– Anxiety in the sense of existential fear – inability to cope with fear

With the progression of the personality changes hyper-, hypo- and heterotypical personality features develop.

Mental rigidity and indecisiveness are leading characteristics of dementing personality change.

Differentiation of abnormal personality traits in the context of developing dementia

Pseudoneurasthenia (early signs, frequency 64%)	Impaired concentration and short-term memory Increased autonomic vasomotor disturbances Increased fatigability
Organic personality change (frequency 32%)	*Hypertypical personality development* There is a caricaturing of pre-existing character traits with progressive loss of the ability to compensate (the chatterbox becomes more garrulous, the skinflint more miserly, etc.).
	Hypotypical personality development There is 'flattening' of personality; individuality is progressively lost. Personality moves towards extinction.
	Heterotypical personality development The pathological pocess brings about a complete restructuring of the personality (e.g. bill dodging, cheating, sexual transgression).
Irreversible dementia (frequency 4%)	Impairment and loss of a previously intact personality. Loss of initiative and the ability to perform complex actions. Disintegration of personality.

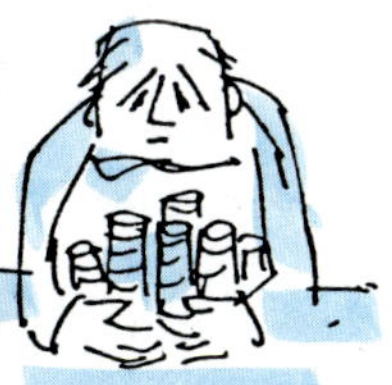

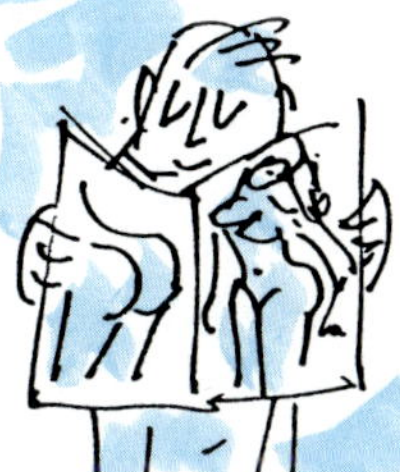

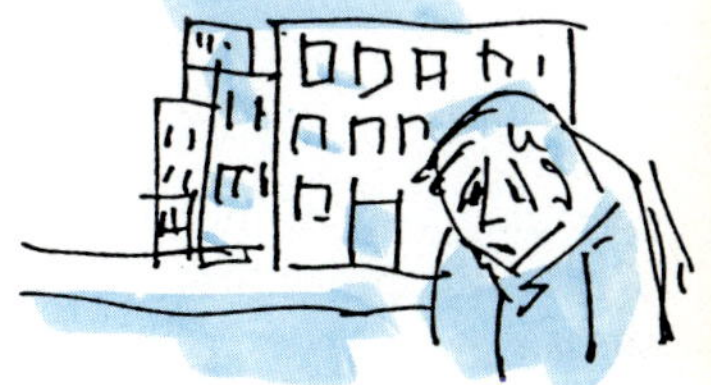

An unstimulating environment of an old people's home results in a fast decline in nerve cell activity and in a loss of physical and mental vitality.

The Patient's History Provides Important Clues in the Assessment of Dementing Personality Loss

When a dementing process is suspected, the diagnostic procedure begins with careful history-taking, which must be *multidimensional* and *followed up at subsequent interviews.* This enables progression to be included as one of the factors in the diagnostic process. As well as the objective assessment by the doctor or psychologist (aimed in particular at detecting cases of reversible dementia), the patient's own subjective assessment is of particular importance as a guide to future treatment.

The patient should address the following questions:

- How does he view his illness?
- What symptoms are caused by it?
- How do these symptoms affect his ability to cope with daily life?
- What does he feel about the future?

The answers to these questions help the doctor to draw up a realistic ability profile for the patient including both positive and negative aspects. Information obtained from the person in closest contact with the patient is also of decisive importance but, despite all the information that can be obtained in such ways, thorough clinical examination is still essential in order to exclude causes of reversible dementia.

The diagnosis of incipient dementia begins with careful history-taking. The diagnostic procedure is multidimensional and extends over several sessions.

Particular importance attaches to self-assessment by the patient and assessment by the person(s) closest to him, as well as to history-taking and clinical examination by the doctor.

Elucidation of the patient's mental (cognitive) ability profile during history-taking is an important step in the identification of early dementia

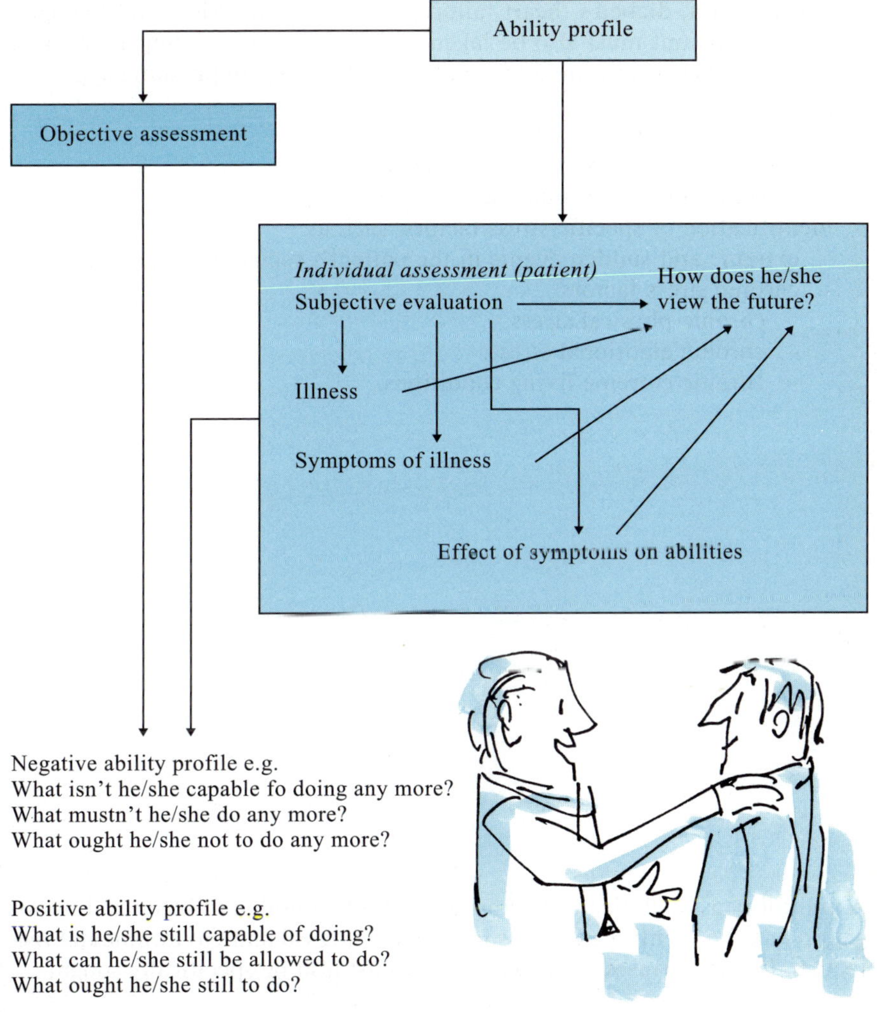

Negative ability profile e.g.
What isn't he/she capable fo doing any more?
What mustn't he/she do any more?
What ought he/she not to do any more?

Positive ability profile e.g.
What is he/she still capable of doing?
What can he/she still be allowed to do?
What ought he/she still to do?

When Early Dementia Is Suspected a Multidimensional Diagnostic Assessment Is Indispensable

The multidimensional assessment of early dementing processes encompasses the following areas:

- identification of psychological, psychometric and neurological irregularities;
- identification of medical risk factors; besides 'normal' risk factors such as hypertension, diabetes, heart failure, blood flow disorders and hypoglycaemia, account must also be taken of factors tending to impede normal recovery, such as insomnia or continual waking (e.g. in prostatic hypertrophy);
- identification of social risk factors;
- identification of psychological risk factors;
- identification of environmental risk factors;
- identification of specific stress factors, such as:
  - extreme and sudden events in the patient's social environment;
  - chronic stress factors:
    - chronic physical stress,
    - chronic emotional stress,
    - chronic extreme living conditions.

A multidimensional diagnostic approach involves both a full clinical investigation and the identification of social, psychological and environmental risk factors. Possible causes of chronic stress must also be specifically sought.

A comprehensive clinical investigation is essential for the diagnosis of early dementia

Neurological and psychiatric investigations
(Paying particular attention to cognitive deficits, emotional disturbances, personality changes, neurological abnormalities, abnormal movement and gait, incontinence, confusional states, depression)

Supplementary neurological investigations
- Electroencephalography (EEG; including sleep EEG, power spectra)
- Electronystagmography
- Computer tomography
- Doppler ultrasound
- Transcranial Doppler ultrasound
- Angiography
- Lumbar puncture
- Magnetic resonance imaging
- (Positron emission tomography)

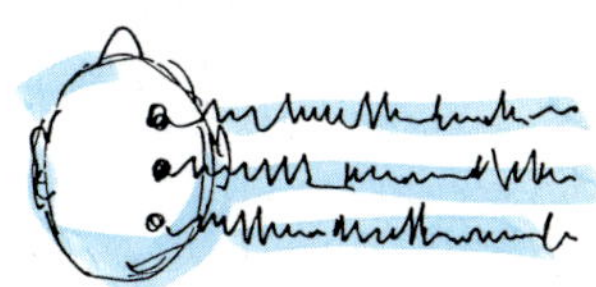

Supplementary medical investigations
- Electrocardiogram (ECG)
- 24-hour ECG
- Standing blood pressure and pulse (e.g. Schellong and de Marée test)
- Echocardiography
- Spirometry

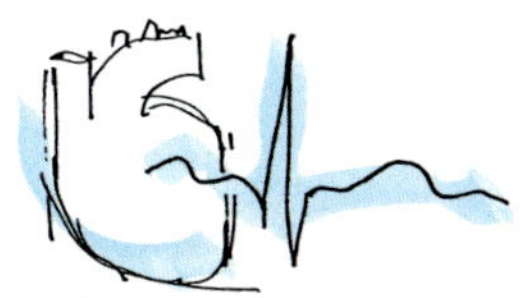

Laboratory investigations
- Haematology: erythrocyte sedimentation rate, haemoglobin, red cell count, platelet count, white cell count, differential count
- Liver function: serum enzymes (GOT, GPT, γ-GT, AP, GLDH), ammonia, serum protein, electrophoresis, prothrombin time
- Kidney function: urinalysis, creatinine
- Metabolism: glucose, cholesterol, triglycerides, high- and low-density lipids, uric acid, vitamin B_{12}, folic acid, thyroid function tests (TSH, T_3, T_4, TRH test), blood gases and pH
- Haemorrheology: haematocrit (optimum for brain 40%), red cell and platelet aggregation, blood and plasma viscosity, red cell elasticity, fibrinogen
- Electrolytes: serum Na^+, K^+, Ca^{++} and Mg^{++}, red and white cell magnesium
- Exclusion of chronic infections: syphilis, AIDS, Borrelia, neurotropic viruses
- Collagen disease
- Drugs: blood levels

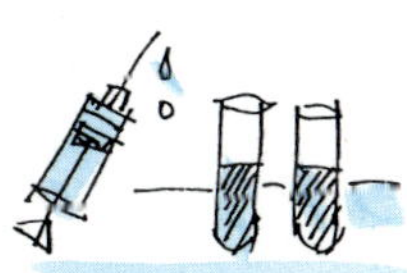

In All Cases of Dementia a Reversible Cause Must First Be Ruled Out

Cognitive impairment is a potential feature of at least 50–60 diseases. Knowledge of which dementing disorders are treatable or improvable demands a high level of differential diagnostic skill. The principal causes of reversible or partially reversible dementia are:

- chronic intoxication (medicines, industrial poisons, narcotics and other habit-forming drugs, alcohol),
- cardiovascular diseases,
- chronic respiratory failure,
- metabolic diseases,
- endocrine diseases,
- vitamin deficiency,
- intracerebral diseases.

Severe depression may also mimic senile dementia. In the USA 40–50% of patients diagnosed as having dementia are in fact suffering form severe depression.

About 60 different disease entities can be associated with dementia-like cognitive impairment, which may therefore respond to treatment of the underlying disorder.

Causes of reversible or partially reversible dementia

Chronic intoxication
Chronic alcoholism: Korsakoff's syndrome
Chronic drug overdosage or misuse: analgesics (containing phenacetin), atropine, scopolamine, barbiturates, digitoxin, disulfiram, fluphenazine, lithium, methotrexate, methyldopa and haloperidol, oral hypoglycaemics, phenothiazines, phenytoin, propranolol, mercurials, steroids, bismuth, etc.
Non-medicinal drugs: heroin, cannabis, amphetamines, etc.
Industrial poisons: organic solvents, including tetrachloroethylene, trichloroethylene and benzene, carbon monoxide and lead poisoning, organic mercury compounds
Endogenous intoxication: hepatic and renal failure, porphyria

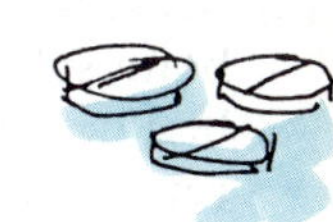

Cardiovascular causes
Long-standing hypertension, ischaemic heart disease, arrhythmias, recurrent asystole, anoxia following successful cardiopulmonary resuscitation, heart failure, cardiomyopathy

Metabolic causes
Chronic malabsorption syndrome, including ileojejunal bypass, malnutrition, hypoglycaemia, hyperlipidaemia, hypoxia (e.g. in sleep apnoea), hyperviscosity, dehydration, disordered electrolytes (e.g. hyponatraemia), hypernatraemia, haemodialysis (16–30 months, progressive encephalopathy, reversible encephalopathy from benzodiazepines)

Chronic respiratory failure,
including sleep apnoea

Endocrine causes
Hypothyroidism (including Fahr's syndrome), thyrotoxicosis, Addison's disease, Cushing's disease, hypo- and hyperparathyroidism, multiple endocrine hypofunction

Vitamin deficiency
Vitamin B_1, vitamin B_6, vitamin B_{12}, folic acid deficiency, pellagra

Intracerebral causes
Subdural haematoma, low-pressure hydrocephalus, subarachnoid haemorrhage, Paget's disease
Inflammatory brain disease: infectious angiitis, neurosyphilis, vasculitis in tuberculosis, fungal infection, sarcoidosis, malaria, septicaemia, general paralysis of the insane, toxoplasmosis
Large meningiomas, acoustic neuroma, cerebral tumours

Primary Degenerative Dementias

Fifty to sixty percent of dementias seen today are dementias of the Alzheimer type. They are regarded as irreversible, although with the aid of modern diagnostic methods other reversible or partially reversible forms of dementia besides multi-infarct dementia are now being diagnosed with increasing frequency.

(1) *Senile dementia of the Alzheimer type* is due either to primary degeneration or to a metabolic cause (idiopathic) leaving cerebral metabolism incapable of maintaining normal brain function.

(2) Irreversible dementias also include *secondary dementias* due to loss of brain substance, for instance in large left-sided cerebral infarcts or cerebral trauma with extensive cortical lesions, or following wide excision of cerebral tumours.

(3) The third primary degenerative brain disease is *parkinsonian dementia.*

(4) The primary irreversible dementing processes also include the *subcortical dementias,* the most important of which are (a) progressive subcortical gliosis (Binswanger's disease), (b) hippocampal dementia and (c) thalamic dementia (disease of the medial thalamic nuclei).

The irreversible dementias include dementia of the Alzheimer type, secondary dementia due to loss of cortical substance, parkinsonian dementia and the subcortical dementias.

Although irreversible dementias become more common with age, the number of reversible dementias also increases

Age-related increase in reversible and irreversible senile dementia

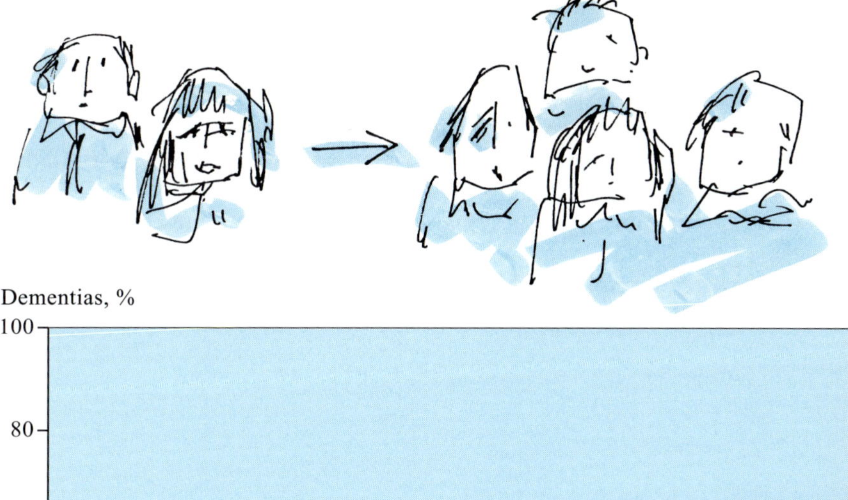

With increasing age there is an increase not only in the incidence of irreversible degenerative dementia but also in the chances of developing a reversible dementia secondary to chronic intoxication, cardiovascular disease, lung disease, metabolic disease or inflammatory brain disease.

The Problem of Psychometric Test Evaluation in Senile Dementia

Once incipient dementia is suspected on clinical grounds, the diagnosis can be confirmed by patient self-assessment, rater assessment, and by tests of cognitive ability. These tests serve to support and verify the diagnosis, they are not a substitute for it. In evaluating individual patients' performances in such tests it is important to bear in mind the experience already gained in the testing of demented patients, since senile dementia follows a specific pattern:

(1) The mental suffering a patient experiences as a result of dementia decreases with the progression of the cerebral dysfunction.
(2) The subjective symptoms are in inverse relation to the severity of the acute brain failure.
(3) After 1, 2 or more years a dementing process culminates in personality loss.
(4) The severity of cerebral dysfunction can be estimated only by comparison with the premorbid state.

Psychometric tests supplement the clinical diagnosis of dementia but are not a substitute for it. The principal instruments used are self-assessment, rater assessment and cognitive ability tests.

The symptoms of senile dementia do not follow a linear course

Relationship between cognitive impairment and subjective well-being in acute organic brain syndrome

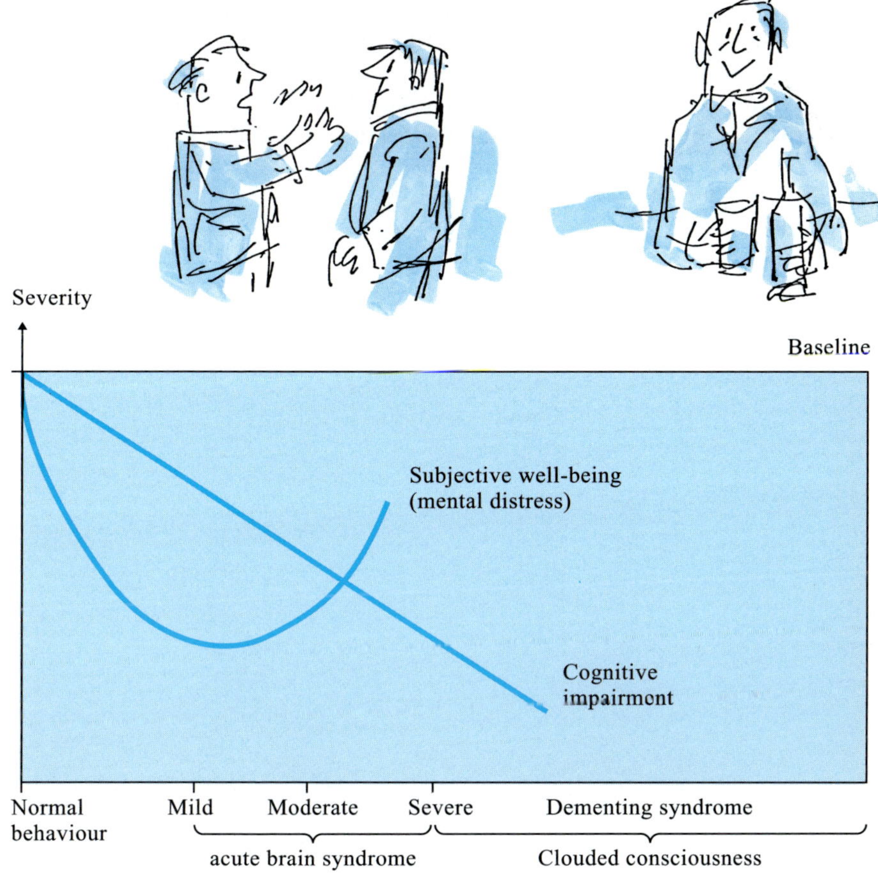

The subjective symptoms exhibited by the patient (mental distress) do not follow a parallel course to the severity of the dementing process. Intellectual deterioration causes the patient much more distress in the initial phases than in the more advanced stages of the disease.

Use of a Psychometric Test Programme in the Differential Diagnosis of Early Dementia

A psychometric test programme enables the doctor to confirm the diagnosis of early dementia, to assess the therapeutic options and to exclude depression. It also provides a basis for monitoring future developments in the patient's condition.
For this only a few easily administered tests are required, such as the Multiple Choice Vocabulary Test (MWT-A/B), the Cerebral Insufficiency Test, the Cerebral Insufficiency Scale (see p. 79), the Dementia-Pseudodementia Differentiation Sheet (DPD, see p. 81), the short form of Hachinski's Ischaemia Scale (S-HIS, see p. 85) and the Short General Intelligence Test (see p. 83).

A psychometric test programme allows dementia of the Alzheimer type (DAT) to be differentiated from multi-infarct dementia (MID). It can also be used to monitor changes in the patient's condition.

A psychometric test programme as an aid to diagnosis in suspected dementia

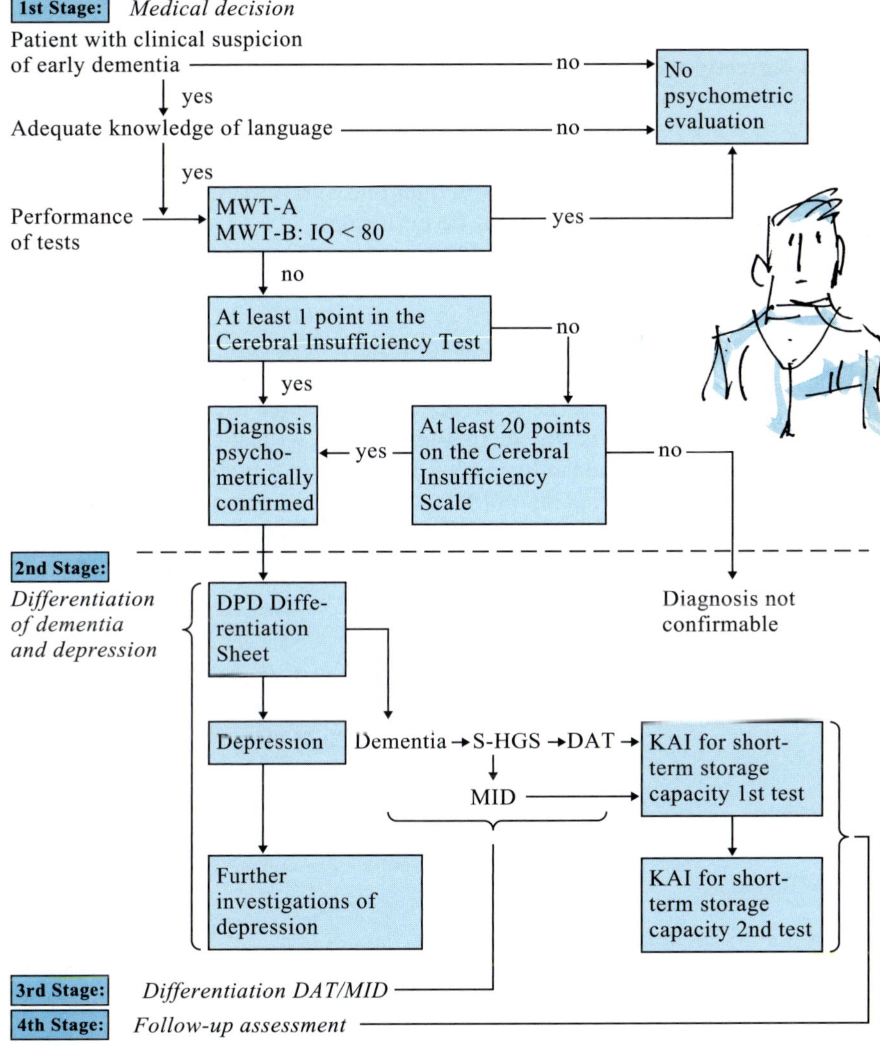

Multiple-Choice Vocabulary Test and Cerebral Insufficiency Test for the Exclusion of Senile Dementia

The *Multiple-Choice Vocabulary Test* serves as a check on the reliability of subsequent cognitive ability tests and increases their sensitivity by measuring the remaining level of intelligence. It is a self-administration test in which the patient must choose the correct word from a series of groups of five. The present intelligence of the subject can be determined from the number of words correctly selected (maximum 37). The reliability of this test increases the lower the patient's intelligence quotient (IQ), i.e. the results are most reliable in the IQ range 80–100.

If the patient's result shows an IQ of over 80, then he is capable of understanding the instructions for the subsequent tests. If his result is under 80, the remainder of the test series cannot be performed.

In the first part of the subsequent *Cerebral Insufficiency Test* the patient is shown a series of symbols in which each symbol appears several times in irregular order. The patient is asked to count as quickly as possible the number of times a particular symbol appears and his performance is timed. In the second part of the test the patient has to read out a sequence of As and Bs in 'reversed order', i.e. where the sequence has A, he must say B, and vice versa. Again the performance is timed. In combination with the patient's age and IQ, the test times provide information on whether the clinical suspicion of early dementia is justified or not. If no points are scored in the Cerebral Insufficiency Test, the *Cerebral Insufficiency Scale* is used. Suspicion of early dementia is hardened if 20 points or more are scored on this scale. The maximum score is 38.

The Multiple-Choice Vocabulary Test, Cerebral Insufficiency Test and Cerebral Insufficiency Scale may be used to exclude or corroborate the diagnosis of early dementia.

Examples of psychometric tests that can be used to exclude or corroborate the diagnosis of suspected early dementia

Extract from the Multiple Choice Vocabulary Test MWT-A

(12) halp – strile – stroll – stralp – strult
(13) sanarium – sentarium – sonasium – sensation – seenestion
(14) parage – bargain – argian – brigon – radum

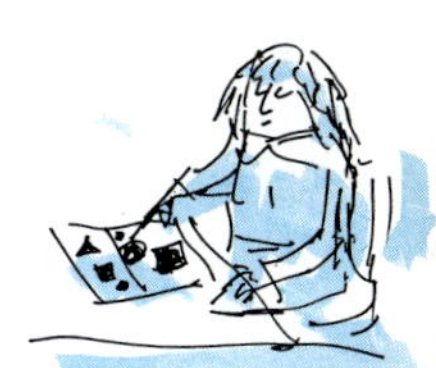

Extract from the Cerebral Insufficiency Test Part I

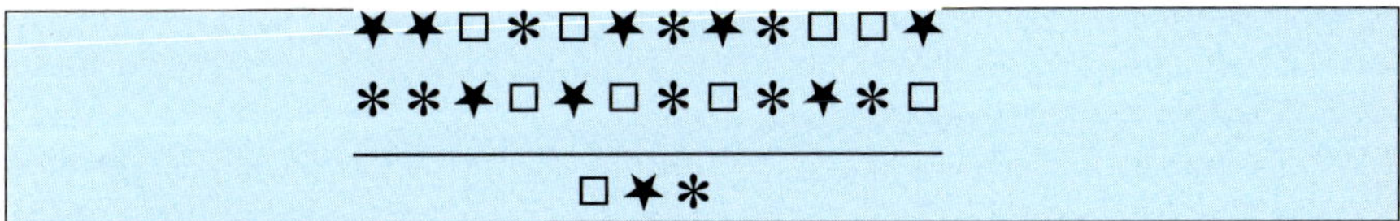

Extract from the Cerebral Insufficiency Test Part II

AABABABBBABAABABA

Extract from the Cerebral Insufficiency Scale

(12) I forget names more often than I used to	yes	no
(13) I forget jobs more often than I used to	no	yes
(14) I make notes more often than I used to so I don't forget things	yes	no
(15) My forehead often feels cold or warm	yes	no
(16) I always feel light-headed in the morning	yes	no
(17) I seem to be yawning a lot recently	no	yes
(18) My nerves are worse than before; little things seem to get me worked up	yes	no
(19) I'm more anxious than before and don't feel as confident about doing things	yes	no

Psychometric Tests for Differentiating between Senile Dementia, Depressive Pseudodementia and Multi-Infarct Dementia

To exclude the possibility of a depression masquerading a so-called pseudodementia, the Dementia-Pseudodementia Differentiation Sheet is employed (see p. 81).
The short form of Hachinski's Ischaemia Scale helps to distinguish multi-infarct dementia from dementia of the Alzheimer type (see p. 85).
Using the Short General Intelligence Test it is possible to follow any progression in the patient's condition and also to monitor the effects of treatment (see p. 81).
Multiplication of the memory span by the information processing speed yields the short-term storage capacity of the brain, which can be expressed as an IQ score.

Early dementia may be characterized with the aid of the Dementia-Pseudodementia Differentiation Sheet and the short form of Hachinski's Ischaemia Scale. The Short General Intelligence Test can be used to follow the evolution of the condition and monitor the patient's response to treatment.

Extract from the Dementia-Pseudodementia Differentiation Sheet

Short psychometric test for the differential diagnosis of depression and senile dementia (to be conducted by doctor):

Name:	Date of birth:	Sex (m/f):	Date:	
Please underline applicable answer			I	II
'Can you tell me what date it is today'? (to within 2 days)			right	wrong
'What is the name of the prime minister?'			right	wrong
'Do you know the name of the street we are in here?' (In cities part of town will suffice)			right	wrong
'Please try and remember the word "exit".'				
'Do you feel much worse in the mornings than in the evenings?'			yes	no
'Do you tend to brood?'			yes	no
'Have you ever had similar complaints in the past?'			yes	no
'Do you feel refreshed after sleep?'			no	yes

More answers in column I suggests depression, in column II suggests dementia.

Assessment of the severity of senile dementia

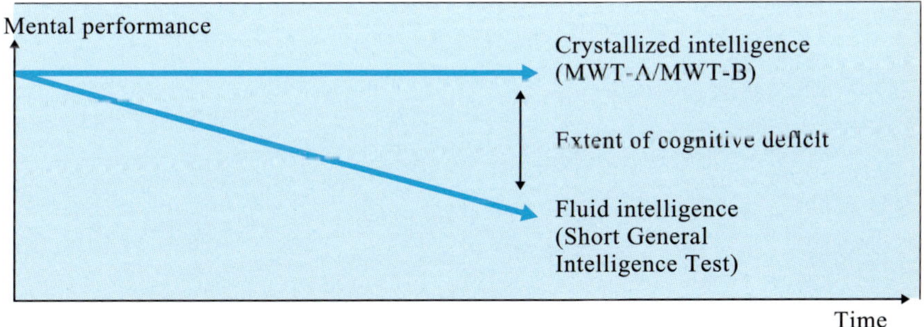

The difference between the IQ scores in the Multiple-Choice Vocabulary Test (MWT-A/MWT-B = premorbid intelligence level) and the Short General Intelligence Test (information processing speed = fluid intelligence) indicates the maximum extent of the intellectual (cognitive) deficit to be overcome.

Psychometric Test for Monitoring the Progression of Senile Dementia and Assessing the Relevance of the Chosen Mode of Treatment

The best test for this purpose is the Short General Intelligence Test, which can also be used to assess the efficacy of treatment. It involves ascertaining the subject's basic information processing factor by measuring the speed with which he can read a sequence of 20 randomly arranged letters. To assess the memory span, the examiner reads out a series of letters or numbers at a rate of one per second and then sees how many the subject can repeat.

The test is relatively simple, takes little time to complete and can even be conducted by an assistant. The difference in IQ score between the Multiple-Choice Vocabulary Test (MWT-A or MWT-B, see p. 79) and the Short General Intelligence Test shows the maximum extent of the cognitive deficit to be overcome.

The Multiple-Choice Vocabulary Test is a measure of crystallized intelligence, while the General Intelligence Test, which is based on information processing speed, is a measure of fluid intelligence.

The test to determine information processing speed measures the level of general intelligence. It is therefore suitable both for monitoring the progression of senile dementia and for studying the efficacy of the treatment selected.

Psychometric test for determining information processing speed

(form translated from German original)

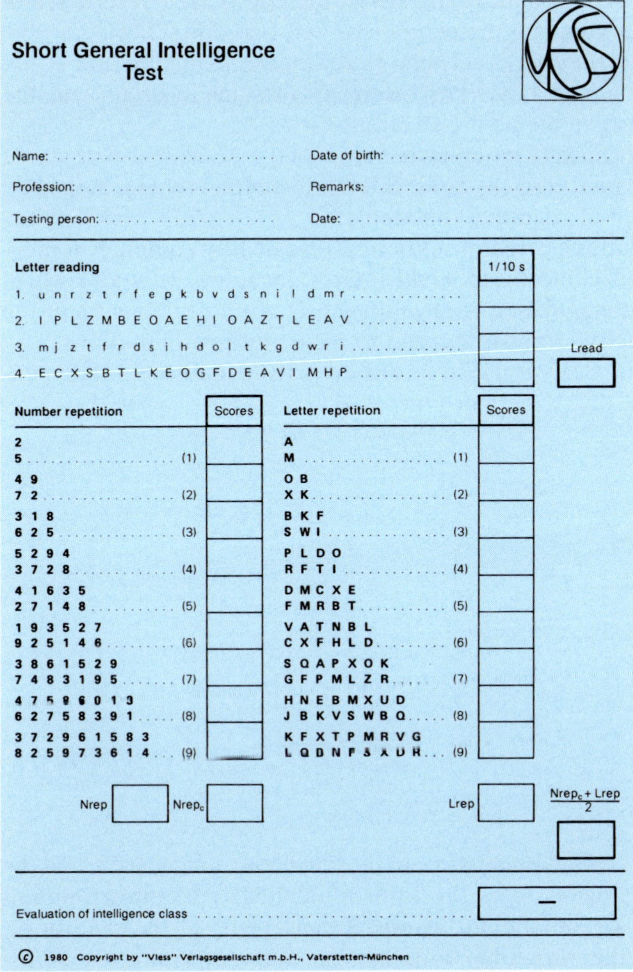

Short General Intelligence Test

Name: .... Date of birth: ....

Profession: .... Remarks: ....

Testing person: .... Date: ....

Letter reading — 1/10 s

1. u n r z t r f e p k b v d s n i l d m r ....
2. I P L Z M B E O A E H I O A Z T L E A V ....
3. m j z t f r d s i h d o l t k g d w r i ....
4. E C X S B T L K E O G F D E A V I M H P ....

Lread

Number repetition		Scores	Letter repetition		Scores
2 5	(1)		A M	(1)	
4 9 7 2	(2)		O B X K	(2)	
3 1 8 6 2 5	(3)		B K F S W I	(3)	
5 2 9 4 3 7 2 8	(4)		P L D O R F T I	(4)	
4 1 6 3 5 2 7 1 4 8	(5)		D M C X E F M R B T	(5)	
1 9 3 5 2 7 9 2 5 1 4 6	(6)		V A T N B L C X F H L D	(6)	
3 8 6 1 5 2 9 7 4 8 3 1 9 5	(7)		S Q A P X O K G F P M L Z R	(7)	
4 7 5 8 6 0 1 3 6 2 7 5 8 3 9 1	(8)		H N E B M X U D J B K V S W B Q	(8)	
3 7 2 9 6 1 5 8 3 8 2 5 9 7 3 6 1 4	(9)		K F X T P M R V G L Q D N F S X U R	(9)	

Nrep $Nrep_c$ Lrep

$\frac{Nrep_c + Lrep}{2}$

Evaluation of intelligence class .... –

IQ score in Multiple-Choice Vocabulary Test minus IQ score in Short General Intelligence Test.

Differential Diagnosis of Moderately Severe and Severe Senile Dementia

In unequivocal cases of senile dementia meeting the diagnostic criteria of DSM III, the Mini Mental State Examination devised by Folstein et al. and the short dementia syndrome test (p. 85) can be used to gauge the severity of the condition and plot its evolution. However, these tests are not sufficiently sensitive for patients with early dementia (see vol. 1 of this series).

Cases of senile dementia divide between multi-infarct dementia and senile dementia of the Alzheimer type. The former is vascular in origin and the latter due to degenerative metabolic changes.

Usually the mental incapacity in senile dementia of the Alzheimer type shows a continuous progression, whereas multi-infarct dementia is characterized by stepwise deterioration of cognitive function.

Not every case of multiple cerebral infarction revealed by computer tomography manifests itself clinically as multi-infarct dementia. It is also worth noting that many patients with a clinical diagnosis of senile dementia of the Alzheimer type are found at post mortem to have multiple infarctions.

Hachinski's Ischaemia Scale is useful in differentiating multi-infarct dementia from dementia of the Alzheimer type.

Moderately severe to severe dementia can be adequately diagnosed using the DSM III criteria. At these stages the Mini Mental State Examination and short syndrome test are suitable for assessing the severity of the condition. Senile dementia of the Alzheimer type can be differentiated from multi-infarct dementia by means of the short form of Hachinski's Ischaemia Scale.

Test criteria in moderately severe dementia and multi-infarct dementia

Outline of diagnostic criteria for senile dementia according to DSM III

(A) Loss of intellectual abilities (impairment of social and occupational functioning)
(B) Memory impairment
(C) At least one of the following:
  (1) Impairment of abstract thinking (inability to find similarities and differences between related words, difficulty in defining words and concepts, etc.)
  (2) Impaired judgement
  (3) Other disturbances of higher cortical function, such as aphasia (speech impairment), apraxia (inability to perform motor activities), agnosia (failure to recognize or identify objects), difficulty with constructional tasks
  (4) Personality change
(D) No clouding of consciousness

Evaluation: If criteria A–C are met, onset of illness is after the age of 65, onset and progression are very slow, memory impairment predominates, then the senile form of Alzheimer's disease should be diagnosed.

Ischaemia Scale of Hachinski et al. [1975] for the diagnosis of multi-infarct dementia

Feature	Score
(1) Abrupt onset of illness	2
(2) Stepwise deterioration	1
(3) Fluctuating course	2
(4) Nocturnal confusion	1
(5) Personality largely preserved	1
(6) Depression	1
(7) Somatic symptoms	1
(8) Emotional lability	1
(9) History of hypertension	1
(10) History of stroke(s)	2
(11) Evidence of associated atherosclerosis	1
(12) Focal neurological symptoms	2
(13) Focal neurological signs	2

Evaluation: 0–4 points = senile dementia of the Alzheimer type; 5–6 points = mixed forms, equivocal; 7–18 points = multi-infarct dementia.

Treatment Options in Early Senile Dementia

The objective of treatment in early dementia is to preserve and increase the integrity of the patient's biological, psychological and social abilities and, if possible, reduce any deficits. Two complementary approaches are available to achieve this: (1) general management and (2) cerebral activation. Their key elements are briefly outlined below.

General management
- Measures to combat psychological, social, environmental, epochal and economic factors predisposing to premature aging
- Amelioration of particularly stressful situations, such as loneliness, loss of role, social discrimiation
- Reduction of medically treatable risks, including withdrawal of drugs with a possible negative effect on higher mental functions
- Treatment of clinically confirmed diseases
- Treatment of attendant psychiatric symptoms
- Specific psychotherapy as opposed to drug therapy

Cerebral activation therapy
- Treatment with cerebral activator drugs: effective drugs are co-dergocrine mesylate (Hydergine), piracetam and pyritinol
- Physical activity and physiotherapy
- Exercising the brain
- Dietary measures

The four components of cerebral activation are used in combination, the objective being to attain the premorbid level of mental function, in other words, the restoration of competence.

The multifactorial aetiology of early dementia requires a multidimensional therapeutic approach. This holistic approach will continue to guide the direction of future treatment.

The four components of cerebral activation therapy

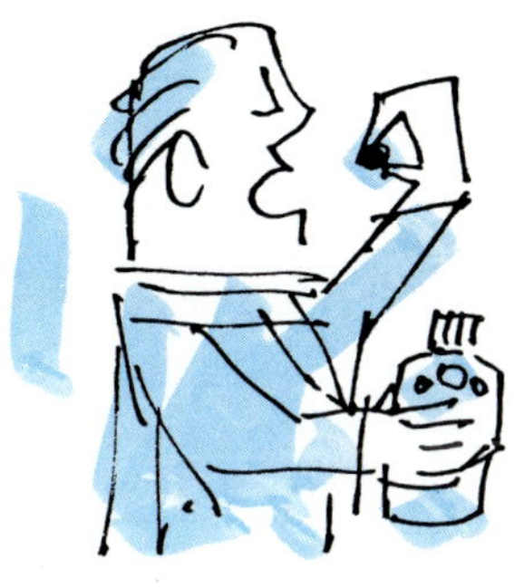

Cerebral activators

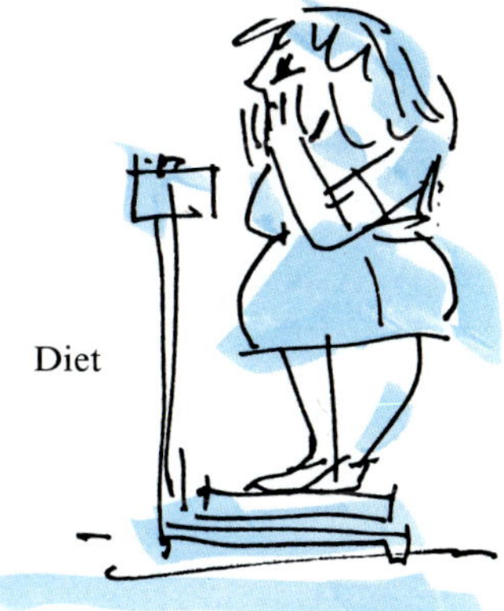

Diet

Physical activity

Brain training

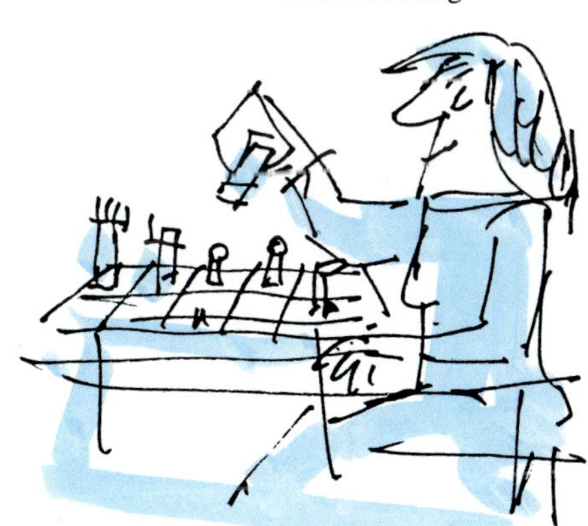

Senile Dementia and Multi-Infarct Dementia

P. Slater

Aging Is the Greatest Predisposing Factor for Dementia

The great majority of dementias are diagnosed as either senile dementia of the Alzheimer type or multi-infarct dementia. The probable predisposing factor for these conditions, as far as they are known, is aging. Dementia is not simply caused by 'senility', but affects mainly the elderly.

The incidence of senile dementia of the Alzheimer type increases exponentially with age. There are only isolated cases below about 45 years of age, which are called presenile dementia (Alzheimer's disease), first described in 1906 by Alois Alzheimer. The incidence of senile dementia of the Alzheimer type begins to increase steeply in the age range 65–75 years. Although estimates vary, it is claimed that 4–5% elderly people may be affected by dementia and almost all of them are in the older age brackets.

The average age of populations in Western Europe is tending to increase. The aging of populations world-wide has automatically led to an increase in the number of persons at risk of dementia. However, despite these gloomy predictions, it has to be remembered that 80% of people over the age of 80 are not demented.

Senile dementia is definitely a disease of the elderly. Aging is the clearest and strongest predisposing factor for developing dementia.

Estimating the incidence of the main age-related dementias

Approximate relative prevalence of different types of dementia

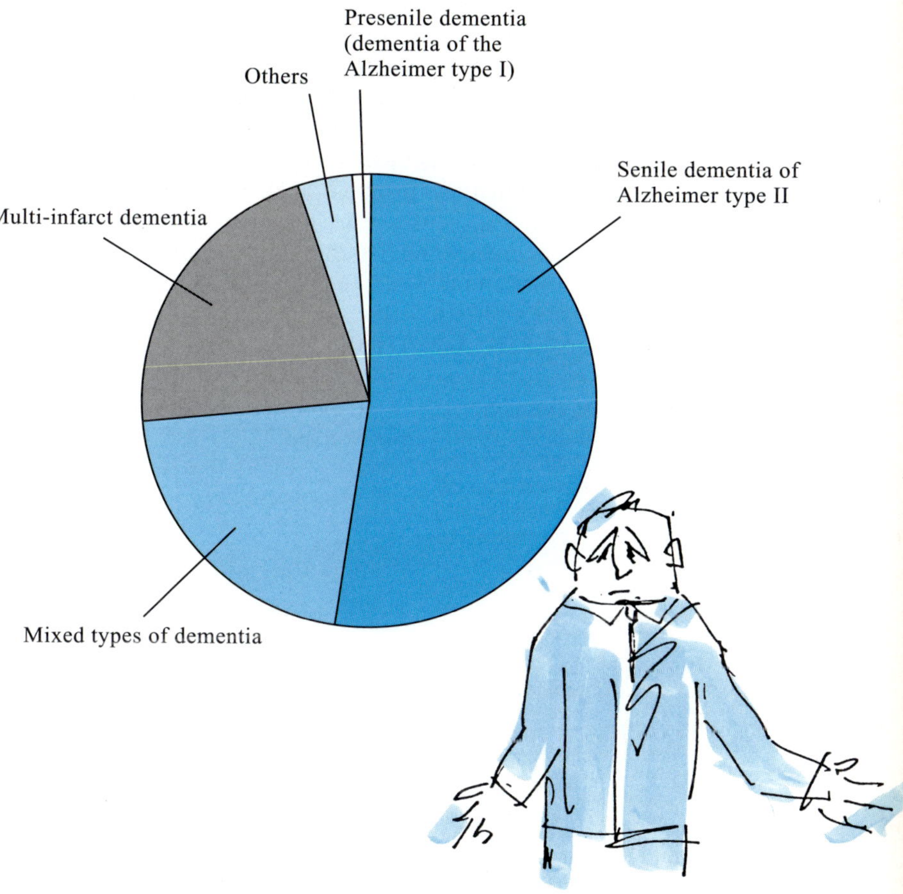

The incidence of dementia is estimated at about 5% for persons over the age of 65, rising to >20% for the population of over 80. More than 50% of demented old people suffer from a primary degenerative dementia (mostly senile dementia of the Alzheimer type II) and about 25% have vascular or so-called multi-infarct dementia, or a mixture of Alzheimer's disease with multi-infarct dementia.

The Risk for Presenile Dementia Is Inheritance

In 1906 Alois Alzheimer reported about a primary degenerating dementing brain disease in persons being in the middle of the 40s. This presenile dementia was called Alzheimer's disease.
Of the major psychiatric illnesses, Alzheimer's disease has received the most attention from geneticists. Inherited, or familial, Alzheimer's disease was first recognized in a few families; later it was more widely recognized. It is accepted that in a minority of cases Alzheimer's disease is inherited as an autosomal-dominant disorder, spreading over several generations.
Familial Alzheimer's disease has an early onset with the first symptoms in the 5th or 6th decade of life and a relentless progression of the disease. Just how many cases of early-onset Alzheimer's disease are inherited is not known, but a family history of dementia increases the likelihood of a familial condition. Also, there is some suggestion of an increased incidence of Down's syndrome among relatives of Alzheimer's disease cases. In families with Alzheimer's disease only some members of the family develop conditions of a presenile dementia. Advanced age of the mother is also a well-known risk for Down's syndrome and, because of the genetic link of the offspring developing Alzheimer's disease late in life, this is not a proven fact.

A family history of presenile dementia or Down's syndrome is a firmly established risk factor for Alzheimer's disease. It must be assumed that the great majority of old-age Alzheimer's disease cases are not inherited.

How great is the risk of developing an inherited presenile dementia?

An inheritance risk factor for Alzheimer's disease implies that the relatives of those afflicted with the familial form of the disease are themselves at some risk, but deciding how great is the risk is guesswork. An increased inheritance of the disease in family members of those with confirmed Alzheimer's disease has only occasionally been reported.

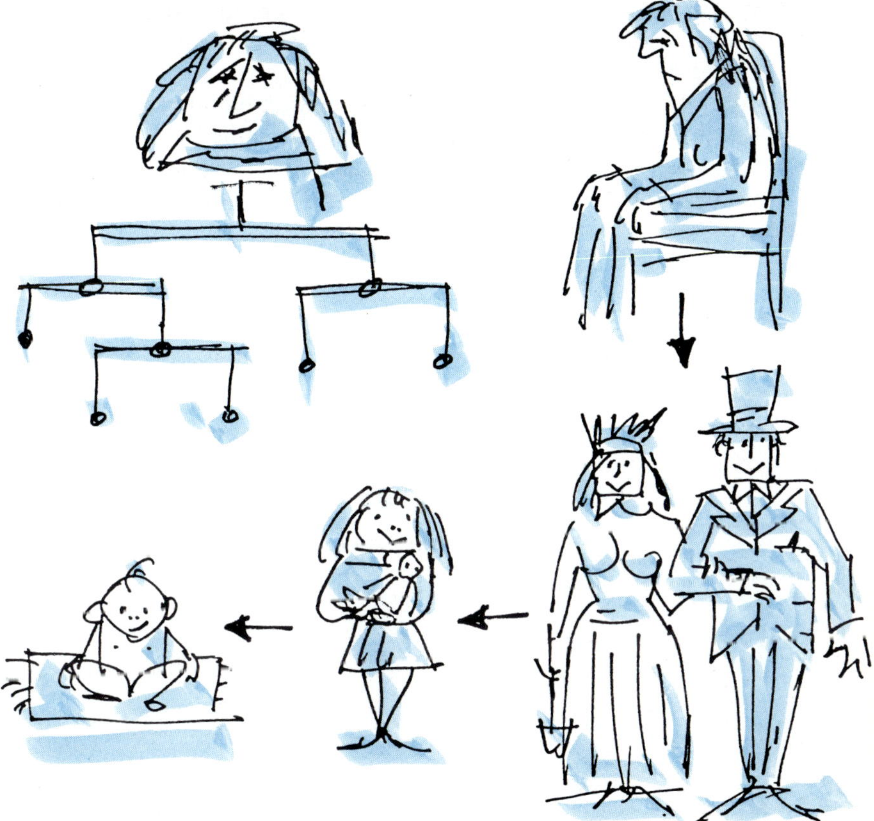

Early testing for Alzheimer's disease
No attempt has been made to develop a gene test for presymptomatic testing for familial Alzheimer's disease. In the absence of any effective treatment to combat the disease, eugenic testing is probably not justified at the present time.

Chromosomal Abnormalities Are Responsible for Familial Presenile Dementia (Alzheimer's Disease)

The particular chromosome affected in familial Alzheimer's disease is the same responsible in Down's syndrome (trisomy 21). Individuals suffering from Down's syndrome who survive into middle age invariably begin to show a loss of acquired skills coincident with the onset of dementia. Post-mortem brains from demented Down's subjects dying at later ages (>40) have the classic pathology of Alzheimer's disease, together with the same neurochemical deficits. The association between Down's syndrome and Alzheimer's disease led to a successful investigation of the gene defect in familial Alzheimer's disease, which was located on chromosome 21.

The gene for the β-amyloid protein found in cerebral blood vessels and the plaques of Alzheimer's disease was traced to chromosome 21.

It appears that not all familial cases are linked to the chromosome 21 site, which raises the possibility of genetic heterogeneity in familial Alzheimer's disease.

A gene fault on chromosome 21 is responsible for familial Alzheimer's disease. Those with Down's syndrome (trisomy 21) invariably develop brain abnormalities characteristic of Alzheimer's disease in later life.

The abnormal gene that causes familial presenile dementia

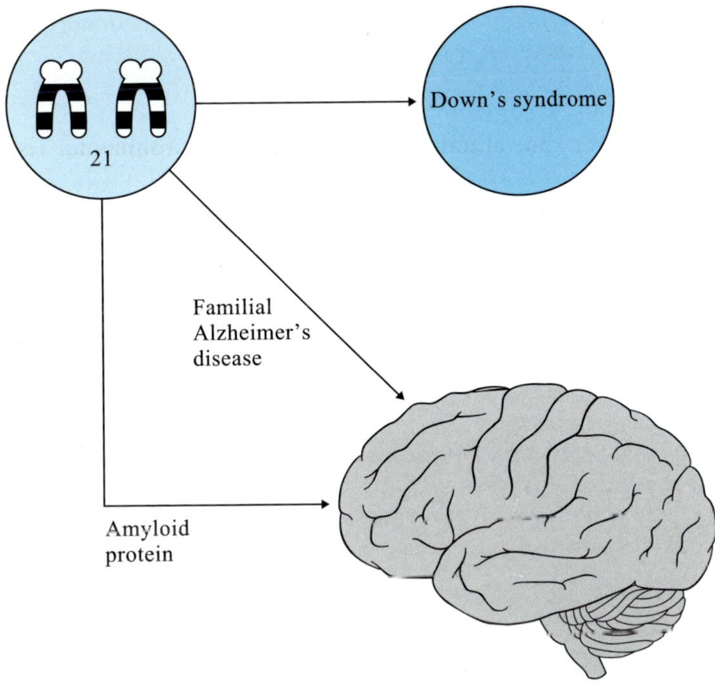

There are abnormal genes on chromosome 21 which produce amyloid in the brain, which turns up in senile plaque cores and small blood vessels, causing familial Alzheimer's disease.

Are Environmental Factors a Risk for a Dementing Brain Disease of the Alzheimer Type?

Theories about the cause of Alzheimer's disease have included metabolic abnormalities, loss of trophic factors, infectious agents and toxins.

Infectious Agents
There is no evidence that a senile dementia of the Alzheimer type is transmissible. All attempts to infect monkeys with the disease have failed. Infectious agents (slow viruses, prions) thought to be responsible for some rare dementias like Creutzfeldt-Jakob's disease (spongiform encephalopathy) or kuru disease seem to be ruled out as the cause of Alzheimer's disease.

Aluminium and Alzheimer's Disease
Some researchers believe that aluminium is a suspect environmental risk factor for Alzheimer's disease. This is a controversial topic and much of the evidence linking aluminium, or other metals, with senile dementia of the Alzheimer type is only circumstantial. The facts are:
(1) Aluminium in the form of aluminosilicates is concentrated in cells that contain neurofibrillary tangles and in the amyloid cores of senile plaques of persons with Alzheimer's disease.
(2) Aluminium is neurotoxic. In some species of animal, aluminium can produce neurofibrillary degeneration, although not the same as Alzheimer type tangles. Dialysis encephalopathy, which is recognized clinically by bone damage, neurological signs, dementia and/or loss of memory and slowing of the EEG, is a well-recognized consequence of renal dialysis carried out with water containing aluminium oxide. It is preventable and removing most of the aluminium oxide from the water reduces the risk of dialysis encephalopathy.

Although infectious agents are ruled out as the cause of a dementing brain disease of the Alzheimer type, the debate about aluminium toxicity continues. There are unsolved questions about aluminium; it is open if the proven presence of the metal in the brains of subjects with senile dementia is related to neurodegeneration, in particular if it is cause or effect.

Does aluminium in drinking water pose a risk for a dementing brain disease of the Alzheimer type?

Geographical surveys have suggested that there might be a link between the amount of aluminium silicates in drinking water and cases of senile dementia of the Alzheimer type. The incidence of senile dementia of the Alzheimer type in Great Britain was above average in areas where the water supply contained relatively high levels of aluminium. However, it has to be remembered that the water supply only accounts for a small proportion of aluminium intake, and most aluminium ingested comes from food (tea, some fruit juices and cake mixes etc.). Aluminium is the second most frequent element – after silicium – in our environment.

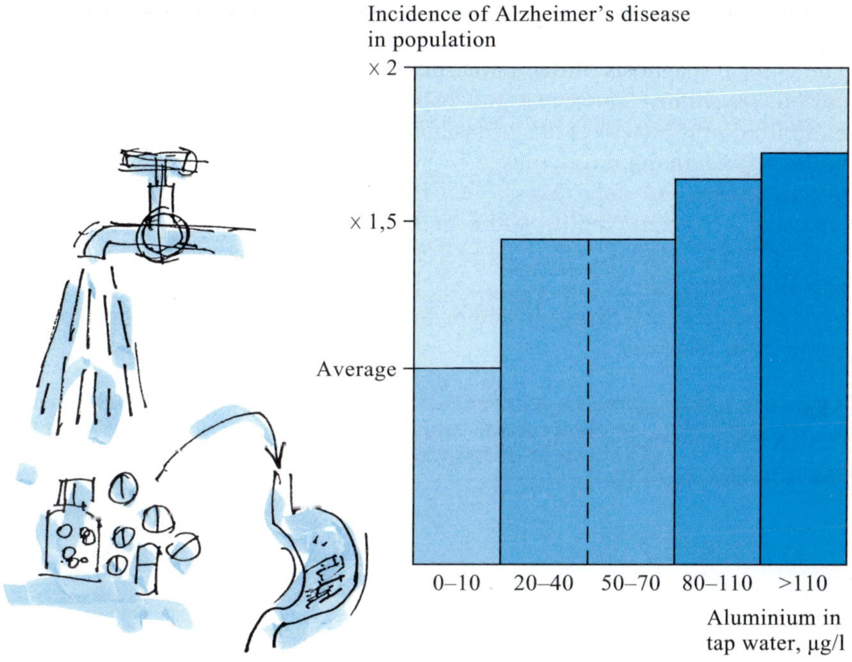

Some medicines contain aluminium
Aluminium salts have long been an ingredient of many medicines, mainly antacids used to treat dyspepsia. There is no evidence that this poses a risk for developing a dementing brain disease.

How to Make a Clinical Diagnosis of Dementia

Dementia is a syndrome which develops over several months. Early symptoms of dementia are usually mild and insidious. Often the symptoms (e.g. memory loss) have developed for some time before the patient or a relative decides that something is wrong.

The first step is to establish that the patient really has a dementia of the Alzheimer type and is not presenting with signs and symptoms of a condition that is masquerading as dementia. Depression, confusional states and 'benign forgetfulness of old age' can all mislead those involved.

Clinical Examination

Dementia is diagnosed by clinical examination with the aid of psychometric testing. The principal characteristics of dementia have been used to define criteria for diagnosis (e.g. DSM III).

The clinical diagnosis of dementia includes: medical history, clinical examination, psychiatric interview and psychometric testing. Mini Mental State Examination [Folstein et al.: J Psychiat Res 1975;12:189–198; the questionnaire is given in detail in volume 1 of this series] is performed with a simple questionnaire and only takes a few minutes. Questions to probe memory, language, arithmetic ability and orientation are included.

The opinions of close relatives are especially important; the extent of the cognitive impairment may be more apparent to others. Facts about addiction to or dependence on drugs (whether prescribed or not) and alcohol may also come from relatives.

Neuropsychological Testing

A specialist neuropsychological assessment should be arranged if clinical examination suggests dementia.

Clinical examination and psychometric testing are needed for diagnosis of dementia.

Practical tests to establish a dementing brain disease

Criteria used to diagnose dementia

(1) Cognitive impairment
(2) History of deterioration of memory and other cognitive functions
(3) Wide-ranging cognitive problem rather than focal
(4) No impairment of consciousness or alertness; any clouding of consciousness prevents a diagnosis of dementia

Diagnosis of dementia according to the Diagnostic and Statistical Manual (DSM III revised) of the American Psychiatric Association [1987]

(1) Evidence of short- and long-term memory impairment
(2) At least one of the symptoms must be present:
   - impairment of abstract thinking
   - inability to find similarities and differences between related words
   - difficulty in defining words and concepts
   - impaired judgement
   - disturbances of higher cortical function, such as aphasia, apraxia, agnosia, inability to copy three-dimensional figures etc.
   - personality change
(3) Items (1) and (2) must interfere with work, social activity or personal relationships
(4) Consciousness must not be clouded (i.e. no delirium)
(5) Either
   - evidence from history, physical examination or laboratory tests of a specific organic factor related aetiologically to the disturbance or
   - absence of non-organic mental disorder, such as depression

Dementia can be graded:

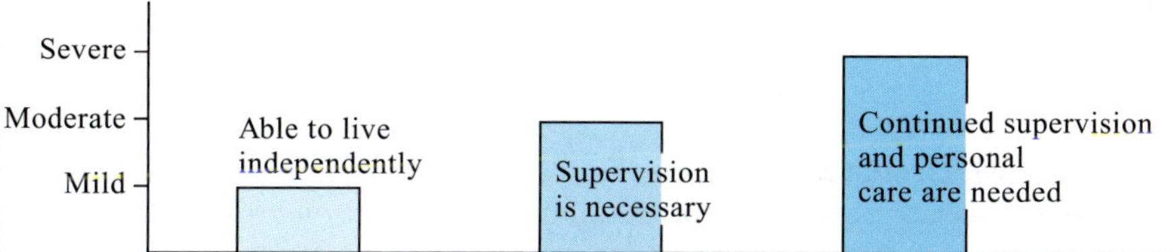

Differential Diagnosis of Subcortical and Cortical Dementias

If laboratory tests fail to show metabolic, hormonal or toxic causes for the dementia, the possibilities of vascular, subcortical or degenerative dementias have to be considered.

Two important clinical features of any dementia that help in differential diagnosis are: (1) the nature of the onset and the progression of the symptoms, (2) the presence or absence of neurological signs and symptoms that can be attributed to a focal lesion.

Subcortical Dementias

The term subcortical dementia was first applied to the cognitive impairment of progressive supranuclear palsy. This is characterized by memory loss and personality changes, plus a striking slowness in making verbal responses in a co-operative individual with no other communication difficulties. Association cortex problems (aphasia, agnosia and apraxia) are noticeably absent. Generally, subcortical dementia describes brain diseases with a clinical picture of movement disorders with dementia, apathy, slowness in responding but no cortical features, and includes normal-pressure hydrocephalus, Parkinson's disease with dementia and Huntington's disease.

Cortical Dementias

Presenile dementia (Alzheimer's disease, Pick's disease) and multi-infarct dementia are examples of cortical dementias. There is much cortical pathology in Alzheimer's disease, inducing aphasia, agnosia and apraxia. Neurological signs, which indicate damage to the basal ganglia and other subcortical structures, appear only in advanced forms of Alzheimer's disease.

The use of the term subcortical to distinguish the dementias associated with Parkinson's disease etc. from Alzheimer's disease has been criticized because both conditions involve degeneration of cortex and subcortical structures.

Multi-infarct dementia can span the borderline between cortical and subcortical dementias.

One way in which subcortical dementia differs from a cortical dementia like Alzheimer's disease is that the former may present with neurological signs.

How to reach a conclusion about the type of dementia

Dementia diagnosis flow chart

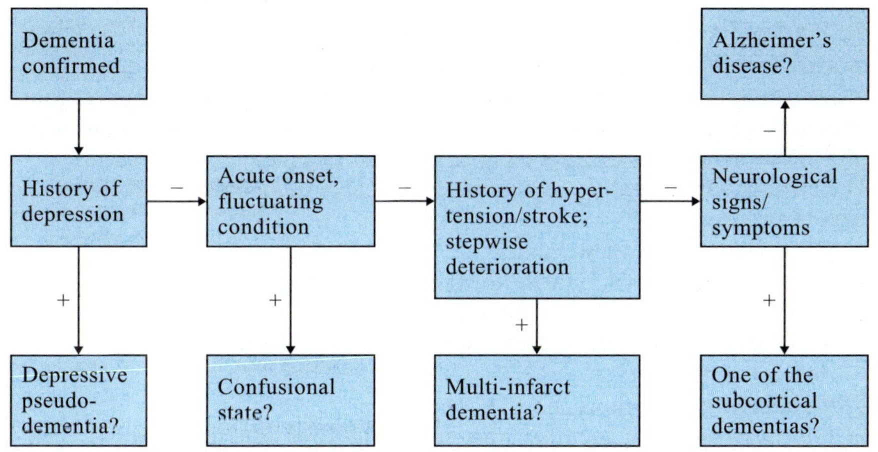

Comparison of subcortical and cortical dementias – main features to look for during clinical examination

Function	Subcortical dementias	Cortical dementias
Mental status		
Language	normal	aphasia
Memory	forgetful, poor retrieval	amnesia, cannot learn new information
Cognition	slowed	severely impaired
Personality	apathetic	unconcerned
Mood	affective disorders	normal
Motor system		
Speech	dysarthric	normal[1]
Posture	abnormal	normal[1]
Movements	slowed	normal[1]
Gait	abnormal	normal[1]

[1] Motor system may be affected in late stage of Alzheimer's disease.

The Diagnosis of a Dementing Brain Disease of the Alzheimer Type Is a Difficult Task

There are no clinical or laboratory tests that give a definite diagnosis of a dementia of the Alzheimer type, except for cortical biopsy. Dementia of the Alzheimer type is diagnosed when the nature and course of the dementia fits in with the known pattern of degenerative illness and when no other cause for the dementia can be found. The disease is normally confirmed from a post-mortem pathological examination of the brain, based on numerous neurofibrillary tangles and plaques throughout the cerebral cortex and hippocampus. Sometimes a clinical diagnosis of Alzheimer's disease turns out to be incorrect at autopsy.

The criteria which enable a diagnosis of probable dementia of the Alzheimer type to be made are:

- clinically established dementia;
- no other concurrent illness, hormone imbalance or brain disease which could account for some of the symptoms seen;
- onset after age 40 years (presenile dementia) and most often after 65 (senile dementia);
- deficits in two or more areas of cognition;
- the impairment of memory and other cognitive functions must be progressing.

Aids to the diagnosis of Alzheimer's disease include:

- a progressive deterioration of easily defined cognitive functions such as language (aphasia), motor skills (apraxia) and perception (agnosia);
- problems occurring with daily living and self-care;
- a family history of dementia;
- electroencephalogram normal or with increased slow wave activity.

Dementia of the Alzheimer type is diagnosed from the clinical signs and when no other cause for the dementia can be found. A definite diagnosis needs a brain cortex biopsy or post-mortem autopsy.

Aetiological and pathogenetic heterogeneity of senile dementia needs a good knowledge of the disease

Diagnostic features of multi-infarct and degenerative dementias

Multi-infarct dementia	Degenerative dementia
History of stroke (most significant) and chronic hypertension (secondary importance)	–
–	Family history of dementia (presenile dementia)
Abrupt onset and stepwise deterioration	Insidious onset, slow progression
Focal neurological signs and symptoms early in the condition	–
–	Motor problems (gait disorders, myoclonus) only in advanced disease

Variations in the presentation of a dementing brain disease of the Alzheimer type

Inheritance	sporadic or familial
Course of disease	rapid progression slow progression
Age of onset	presenile (40–55 years) senile (> 65 years)
Motor deficits (usually late stage)	none extrapyramidal problems myoclonus
Brain hypometabolism	parietal and temporal lobes frontal lobes (decreased glucose turnover measured with positron emission tomography)

Dementia of the Alzheimer Type, Its Course and Prognosis

Presenile (Alzheimer's disease) and senile dementia are characterized by a progressive neurodegenerative condition that once started never stops. The striking clinical feature of dementia of the Alzheimer type, in the early stages, spares the visual, sensory and motor systems. Memory loss is the most prominent sign and symptom, coupled with the inability to learn new information (amnesia). Visuospatial problems, such as getting lost in familiar territory, are another early symptom. These are the sort of symptoms that cause the patient to seek medical advice. Language, which is badly affected, is where the progression of the disease is especially noticeable. At first, certain words are lost and speech is empty but quite fluent; later on, comprehension is destroyed, and in the late stage the patient is largely mute and unable to comprehend. Motor deficits normally occur only in the late stages of Alzheimer's disease.

Presenile dementia (early-onset Alzheimer's disease) is a rare disease under 65. The severity of the dementia can affect survival and has a poor prognosis. Subjects who show myoclonus, extrapyramidal signs or psychosis early in the disease may undergo a more rapid intellectual decline than those who are free of these problems. Some have suggested that myoclonus early on is a predictor of a more aggressive disease course.

Most cases of senile dementia of the Alzheimer type follow a predictable course. When the disease strikes early (presenile dementia), its progression may be rapid. Senile dementia in old age has a much slower progression. Prognosis, however, is always bad.

The different stages of senile dementia of the Alzheimer type

The three phases of senile dementia (> 65 years)

Stage	Cognitive signs/symptoms	Motor signs/symptoms
Early	mild amnesia; visuospatial problems; calculation, insight and judgement are impaired	none
Middle	severe amnesia; language comprehension impaired; speech spared; delusions and agitation common	none
Advanced	subjects become mute, bedridden and incontinent	pyramidal and extrapyramidal signs common

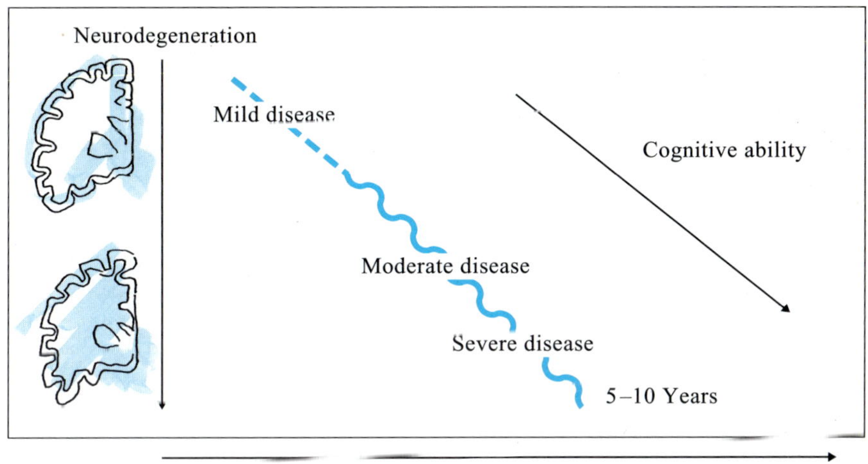

Senile dementia of the Alzheimer type starts in people over the age of 65 years. Patients with senile dementia live for 5–10 years from the onset of symptoms but slow progression with plateaus and survival for 12 or more years are known. Rapid progression with death within 2–5 years is observed mainly in presenile dementia (Alzheimer's disease) with ages between 35 and 55. The incapable, bedridden scenario which all too often is the final stage of Alzheimer's disease is also the killer; bronchopneumonia is given as the immediate cause of death for the majority of patients suffering from senile dementia of the Alzheimer type or presenile dementia.

A Few Dementias Are Reversible

The great majority of dementias turn out to be dementing brain diseases of the Alzheimer type or multi-infarct dementia. Even so, the existence of potentially reversible dementias influences the laboratory investigations that are applied to the diagnosis of dementing diseases. No one knows the true incidence of potentially reversible dementias.
All kinds of medical problems as well as many drugs can give rise to dementia-like states. The brain is susceptible to metabolic disturbances. In such cases, the onset is usually rapid (1–2 days).
The most likely causes of reversible dementia are drug intoxication, depression (pseudodementia), metabolic problems (electrolyte imbalance, exsiccosis) and pulmonary diseases.

Drug Toxicity
The worst drugs prone to cause intellectual impairment, especially in the elderly, are sedatives, hypnotics, tranquillizers, anticholinergics and antihypertensive compounds. A check should be made on recent drug prescribing if a toxic confusional state is suspected. The symptoms normally subside once the drug is removed. Alcohol abuse should not be overlooked as the possible cause of a dementia-like state.

Depression
Some profoundly depressed patients often show overt signs that suggest dementia. These include slowness, apathy, memory loss and disorientation. The onset can be sudden and there is often a personal or family history of depression. True dementia and depression may sometimes coexist.

Drug toxicity and depressive pseudodementia can be mistaken for the early stage of degenerative dementia and therefore must be considered when making a diagnosis.

Some dementias or pseudodementias that can be treated

Major conditions which induce dementia-like syndromes

Vitamin deficiencies	B_{12}, folic acid, thiamine
Endocrine	hypo-, hyperthyroid, hypo-, hyperparathyroid, Cushing's disease etc.
Infection	pneumonia, meningitis, neurosyphilis, encephalitis etc.
Intracranial	tumours, subdural haematoma, normal-pressure hydrocephalus, head trauma etc.
Vascular diseases	strokes, transient ischaemia, cardiac arrhythmia etc.
Electrolyte disturbances, exsiccation etc.	

Remember that intoxication by therapeutic drugs may cause reversible syndromes resembling dementia.

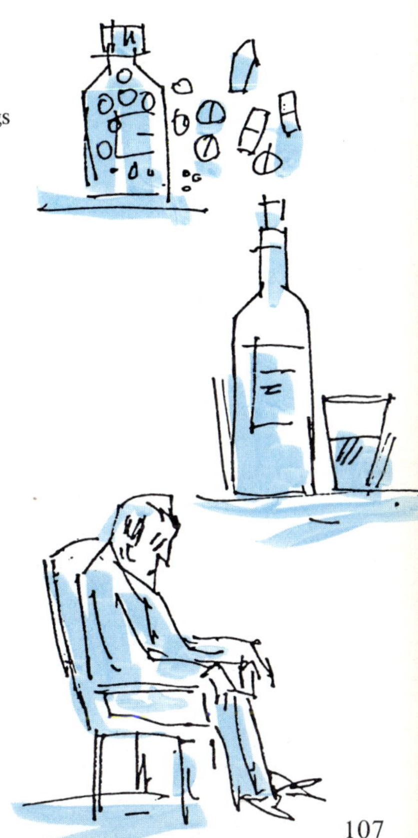

Alcohol abuse is another recognized cause of pseudodementia.

Depression masquerading as dementia can be treated with antidepressant drugs; those with strong anticholinergic properties are best avoided.

Laboratory Tests and Brain Scans That Are Helpful in Searching for the Cause of Dementia

Before a diagnosis of degenerative or multi-infarct (vascular) dementia is considered, it is necessary to show the absence of recognizable illness, hormone imbalance or other brain diseases which could explain some of the symptoms seen and which can be effectively treated.

Very occasionally symptoms of dementia turn out to be hypothyroidism and respond well to appropriate treatment.

Vitamin B_{12} deficiency may cause mental changes without producing any other abnormalities. Red cell folate measurements are made if inadequate diet or megaloblastic anaemia are suspected. Both conditions respond to replacement treatment.

Computer tomography scanning can be a great help in uncovering the cause of some dementing conditions. A scan will pick up lesions (tumours, haematoma), some of which may be treatable, and ventricular enlargement, suggestive of normal-pressure hydrocephalus. A scan will also show multiple infarcts and white matter lesions, and may reveal cerebral atrophy. However, it is important to remember that sometimes a profound dementia is accompanied by very little visible atrophy. It is important to be aware of the fact that no brain scan can diagnose senile dementia of the Alzheimer type.

In practice, a brain scan is not always available and the very elderly are not always amenable to scanning. The need to carry out a scan should be decided after the normal clinical and psychiatric testing.

The newer technique of magnetic resonance imaging is included, but as yet its value in dementia diagnosis is limited, although it may be more sensitive than computed tomography for detecting white matter lesions.

Use of the appropriate laboratory tests may identify some potentially reversible dementias. An overall impression is not sufficient for the diagnosis of senile dementia.

Which examinations are necessary to exclude a reversible dementing brain disease?

Summary of laboratory tests used in the diagnosis of dementia

Test	Diagnostic value
Full blood count	anaemia and other blood diseases, vitamin deficiency (B_{12}, folate, thiamine), iron deficiency, infections
Erythrocyte sedimentation rate	giant cell arteritis
Blood chemistry	
Urea, electrolytes, glucose, calcium, phosphate	liver and kidney function metabolic disorders, drug interactions
Electrocardiogram	cardiac function
Electroencephalogram	epilepsy, Creutzfeldt-Jakob's and Huntington's diseases
Thyroid function	hyper- or hypothyroidism
Chest X-ray	lung cancer, other lung diseases
Computed tomography	tumours, infarcts, hydrocephalus, atrophy
Magnetic resonance imaging	white matter disease including multiple sclerosis

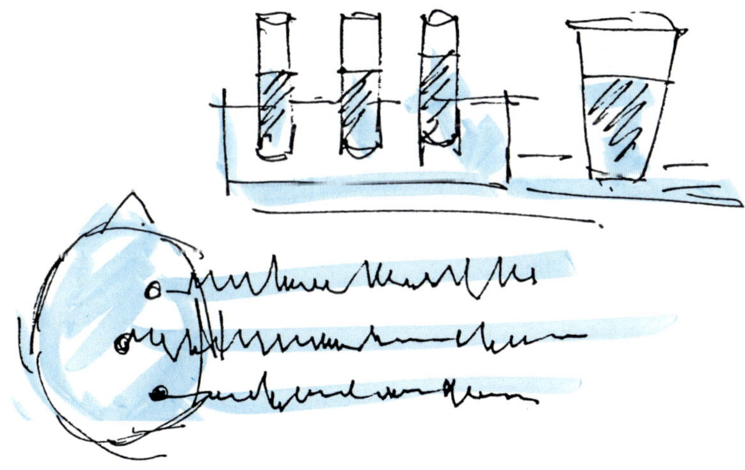

Judicious use of laboratory tests may uncover some potentially treatable cases of dementia.

Multi-Infarct Dementia Causes an Intellectual Decline by Focal Ischaemic Brain Lesions

Multi-infarct dementia is qualitatively similar to the dementias seen in senile dementia, Alzheimer's, Parkinson's disease and other neurodegenerative diseases.

Autopsy studies have shown that 15–20% of elderly patients dying with dementia have extensive areas of cerebral softening (infarcts) with no or little evidence of senile dementia or other types of neurodegeneration. Single photon emission computerized tomography on subjects with multi-infarct dementia shows multiple areas of reduced regional cerebral blood flow corresponding to the infarcts. Also, in the brain areas affected, the autoregulation of cerebral blood flow and normal vasomotor responses may be impaired. Infarcts arise from diseases of extracranial arteries or cerebral arterioles (chronic hypertension not effectively treated). Dementia can result from infarcts that destroy a substantial amount of brain tissue or from small, discrete infarcts that damage areas specifically concerned with memory and cognition.

Binswanger's disease or Binswanger's subcortical arteriosclerotic encephalopathy is a dementing disease clinically similar to multi-infarct dementia, identified by diffuse and patchy cerebral white matter lesions picked up by computer tomography and magnetic resonance imaging. Pathologically, discrete lacunar infarctions are found in the white matter of the internal capsule, thalamus, basal ganglia, cerebellum and elsewhere. The most diagnostic pathology is periventricular demyelination and severe sclerosis of small arteries and arterioles.

Infarcts in the brain can cause a dementia that is similar to the senile dementia of the Alzheimer type. Multi-infarct dementia accounts for 15–20% of all dementias.

The main factors contributing to the development of multiple infarcts in the brain

Four immediate causes of multi-infarct dementia are recognized:
(1) multiple cortical infarcts caused by vascular disease of leptomeningeal vessels (seldom);
(2) multiple small deep (lacunar) infarcts in both hemispheres caused by vascular disease of arterioles; this disease of the cerebral arterioles results mainly from chronic hypertension not effectively treated;
(3) reduced cerebral perfusion by extracranial arterial occlusions;
(4) progressive lesions of the cerebral white matter in Binswanger's disease.

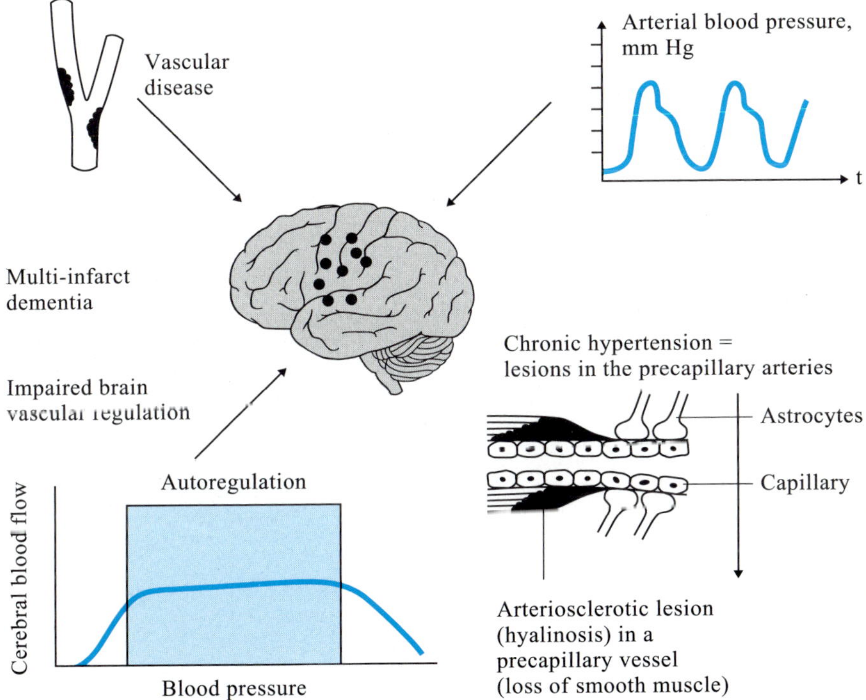

Chronic hypertension, vascular disease, reduced brain blood flow and impaired cerebral vascular regulation are among the most important factors predisposing to brain infarcts.

Differential Diagnosis of Multi-Infarct Dementia

If clinical examination and laboratory tests fail to pinpoint the cause of the dementia, it is advisable to assess the importance of cerebrovascular disease in the pathological process by the use of Hachinski's Ischaemia Scale. A high score on Hachinski's Ischaemia Scale favours a vascular cause for the dementia.

The label of multi-infarct (vascular) dementia is applied whenever there is evidence of vascular disease, stroke, chronic hypertension, and an abrupt onset of the dementia indicating cerebral infarction.

The following key clinical features are usually seen in cases of Binswanger's disease:

- slowly progressive dementia with brief alterations in severity;
- history of chronic hypertension;
- evidence of systemic vascular disease;
- motor signs; especially gait disorders are common.

The dementia has no special characteristics with which to distinguish it from multi-infarct dementia.

Computer Tomographic Scanning

A computer tomographic scan of multi-infarct dementia or Binswanger's disease will reveal any cortical, subcortical and white matter infarcts. However, some caution is needed in interpreting the significance of any revealed brain infarcts. Absolute proof that infarctions of the brain, particularly subcortical lesions, are the cause of the dementia is virtually impossible to obtain. Similar vascular pathologic lesions seen in multi-infarct dementia are often found in the brains of normal individuals. On occasions demented subjects were found to have only mild infarctions. Finally, Alzheimer type pathology and infarcts sometimes coexist, making it difficult to pinpoint the exact cause of the dementia.

The possibility of multi-infarct dementia is evaluated from clinical examination, computer tomography and Hachinski's Ischaemia Scale.

Hachinski's Ischaemia Scale – a valuable tool in the diagnosis of multi-infarct dementia

Hachinski's Ischaemia Scale (differential diagnosis between vascular and degenerative dementia)

	Score
Abrupt onset of cognitive problems	2
Stepwise deterioration	1
Fluctuating course	2
Nocturnal confusion	1
Emotional incontinence	1
History of hypertension	1
History of strokes	2
Evidence of associated atherosclerosis	1
Focal neurological symptoms	2
Focal neurological signs	2

A total score of 4 or less suggests a primary neurodegenerative dementia, whereas a score of 8 or more suggests that the dementia is vascular (multi-infarct) or the mixed type (vascular plus degenerative).

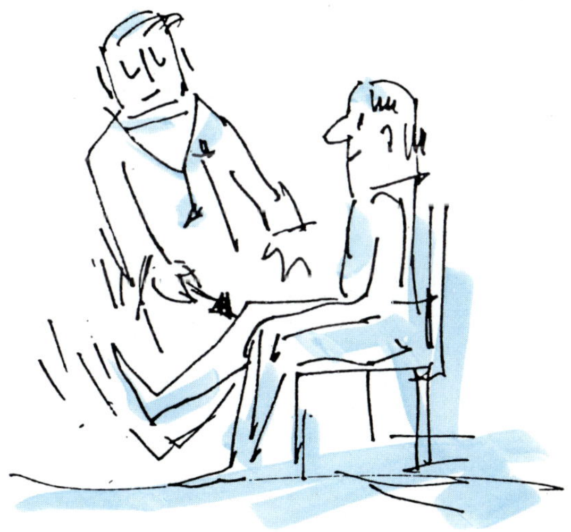

Because the ischaemia score relies on subjective judgements, it is only a guide to differential diagnosis.

What Are the Risk Factors for Multi-Infarct Dementia?

The major risk for developing multi-infarct dementia is untreated chronic hypertension. The vascular disease arising from chronic hypertension is atherosclerosis, which leads to arterial occlusion and subintimal lesions of the smooth muscle by hyalinosis and detritus, which abolishes blood flow autoregulation. The arteriolar disease can produce lacunar infarcts deep in the brain.

Atherosclerosis by itself is not necessarily associated with multi-infarct dementia.

There are other, lesser risk factors for multi-infarct dementia. These are (in order of importance): heart disease, hypercholesterolaemia, cigarette smoking, excess alcohol consumption and diabetes. If one or more of these secondary factors is added to hypertension, the risk of multi-infarct dementia is almost certainly increased.

These factors may increase the risk of brain infarcts by alteri brain perfusion. It is well known that smoking reduces brain blood flow, and studies have shown that the other risk factors can impair regional cerebral blood flow in neurologically normal subjects.

Binswanger's Disease

The precise cause of the white matter lesions seen in Binswanger's disease is unknown. The incidence of radiological features consistent with Binswanger's disease was put at about 1–5% in the elderly, increasing with age, hypertension and severity of cerebrovascular disease. Demyelination of periventricular white matter is a feature of Binswanger's disease.

Chronic hypertension is the major risk factor for multi-infarct dementia.

Hypertension with other risk factors increases the incidence of brain infarcts

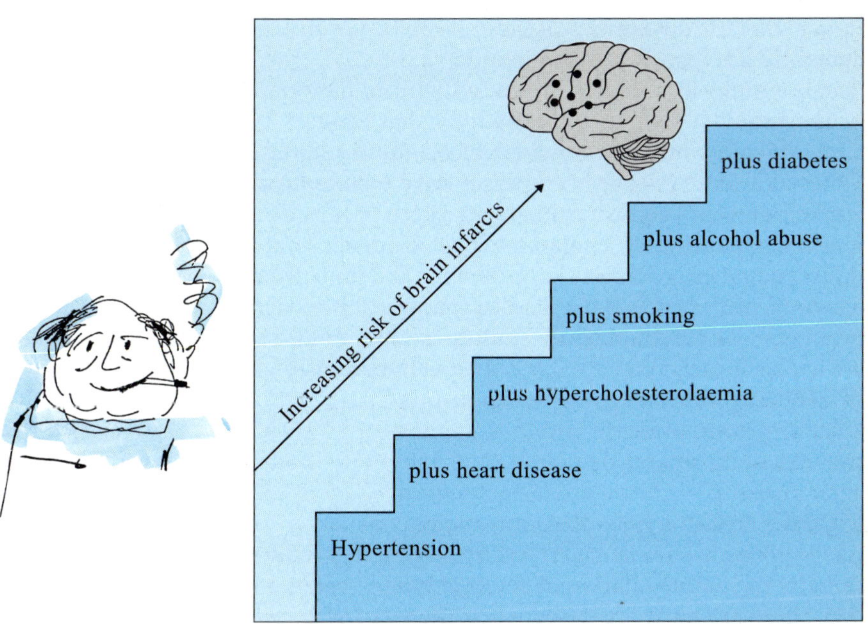

Chronic hypertension
This is the main risk factor for multi-infarct dementia. Other known risk factors for brain infarction are mutually potentiating when combined with chronic hypertension:

(1) *Heavy and chronic drinking*
This reduces brain blood flow and nerve cell metabolism.

(2) *Cigarette smoking*
Nicotine constricts arterioles and slows blood flow.

(3) *Diabetes*
Diabetes mellitus leads to diabetic cerebrovascular disease and predisposes elderly patients to vascular brain lesions.

Can Early Treatment of Risk Factors Reduce the Incidence of Multi-Infarct Dementia?

Strategies for both prevention and treatment of dementias are major health targets. Unfortunately, while the aetiology of senile dementia of the Alzheimer type remains a mystery, it is not possible to identify the risk factors.

In contrast to Alzheimer's disease, some of the risk factors for multi-infarct dementia are recognized and avoidable.

Because multi-infarct dementia results from many small stroke-like episodes in the brain, it follows that anything that reduces the incidence of stroke could have a similar positive effect on multi-infarct dementia. The United States and some European countries have seen reductions in the incidence of stroke in recent years, presumably because of improved treatment for hypertension. Quantitative epidemiological evidence that the number of multi-infarct dementia cases has gone down at the same time is lacking, although it has been suggested that the disease is now less prevalent in some countries. A problem in epidemiological studies is that multi-infarct dementia is not always accurately diagnosed. Control of hypertension is the only rational way of reducing the incidence of multi-infarct dementia. Maintaining in the elderly systolic pressure within a window of 135–150 mm Hg may help to prevent multi-infarct dementia (and the white matter infarcts of Binswanger's disease).

Cigarette smoking is another preventable risk factor for multi-infarct dementia. Smoking a pack of cigarettes or more a day reduces cerebral blood flow, impairs the autoregulation of cerebral blood vessels and increases atherogenesis; these are partly reversed when the smoker gives up this habit.

Control of hypertension reduces the risk of multi-infarct dementia. Cigarette smoking is another avoidable risk.

Drug treatment of hypertension to lessen the risk of multi-infarct dementia

Damage takes place to
the walls of precapillary blood vessels,
particularly arterioles

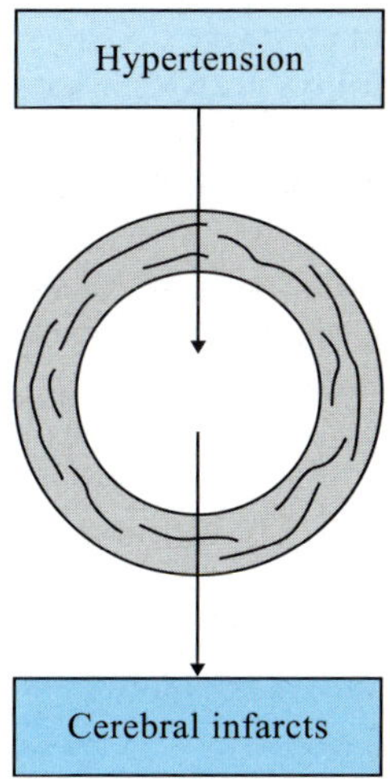

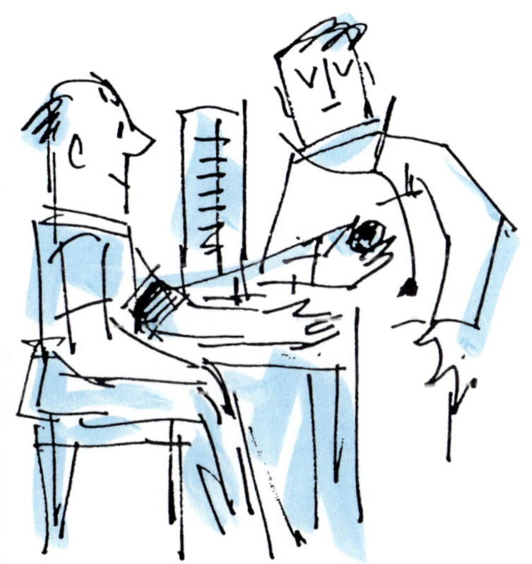

Treatment of elderly hypertensive subjects with blood pressure-lowering drugs should be done cautiously. The aim of treatment should be to slowly and partially bring down the raised arterial pressure. No attempt should be made to quickly normalize the blood pressure because of the danger of impaired cerebral perfusion.

Clinical Course and Prognosis of Multi-Infarct Dementia

Multi-infarct dementia is not the same well-defined neurodegenerative condition as senile dementia. Day-to-day fluctuations in the dementia are seen. The vascular disorders that cause the infarcts of multi-infarct dementia result in stepwise declines with sudden deteriorations in intellect. An interval may follow in which some improvement is seen, but overall the course is downwards.

The severity of the dementia can affect survival in dementia of the Alzheimer type. A severe senile dementia has a poor prognosis. The survival rate of those with multi-infarct dementia is probably worse than in senile dementia. In one study, a 6-year survival rate for subjects diagnosed as having multi-infarct dementia was 12% against an expected survival rate of just over 45%. Another long-term study described a mortality of over 40% during 5 years. The poor prognosis for multi-infarct dementia emphasizes the importance of early detection and primary prevention.

Dementia is not always the immediate cause of death in subjects with multi-infarct dementia; cardiac disease and recurrent strokes are the most frequent causes of death.

The prognosis for multi-infarct dementia is particularly poor. The course of multi-infarct dementia is often one of stepwise deteriorations after an abrupt onset.

The progression of multi-infarct dementia has a characteristic pattern

Repeated brain infarcts which may be cortical or subcortical, cause the dementia.

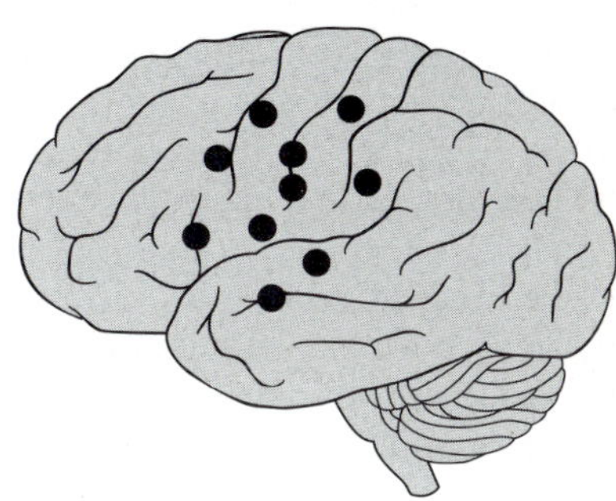

The course of multi-infarct dementia

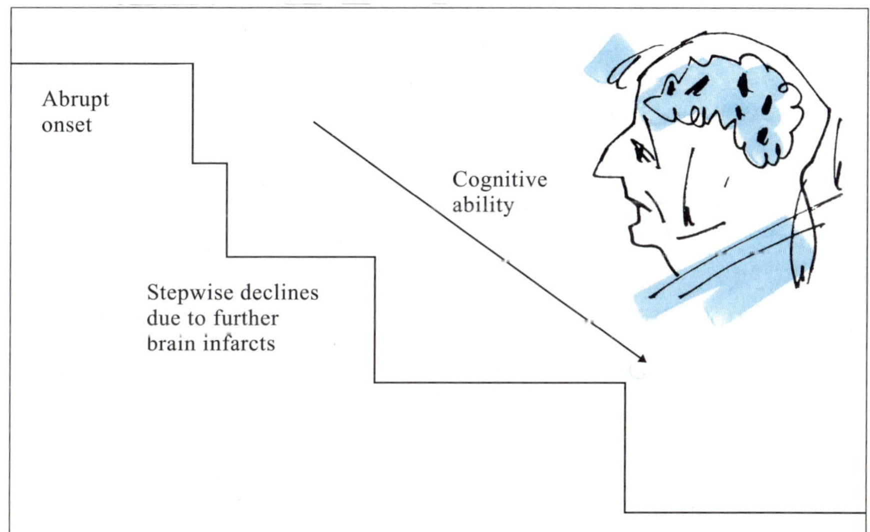

The dementia is correlated with the amount of brain tissue that is damaged or destroyed.

Nootropic Drugs for the Treatment of Vascular and Senile Dementia

Nearly all dementias are caused by neurodegeneration, vascular disease or a mixture of the two. The ideal drug treatment for dementia should be able to:
(a) improve cognition and prevent further intellectual decline in the elderly person with dementia;
(b) prevent further brain damage in multi-infarct dementia;
(c) prevent further neurodegeneration in senile dementia of the Alzheimer type.
Unfortunately it cannot be expected that the various pharmacological and non-pharmacological therapies may compensate irreversible brain lesions. In the past nootropic drugs have only produced some symptomatic benefits in patients with dementia in old age.

Nootropics
The name nootropic literally means drugs that act on the mind. They are recently introduced drugs being evaluated in cognitive impairment. Piracetam is a nootropic prototype.
In experimental animals, nootropics improve some aspects of cognitive performance, usually learning and/or memory, provided that the appropriate tests are used. They also have some protective action on hypoxic brain lesions. Co-dergocrine (Hydergine®) and related compounds proved active and to have remarkably few side-effects, even at large doses.
The results of trials with piracetam and co-dergocrine in senile dementia of the Alzheimer type are, as expected, largely negative, although some mild benefits were claimed when the drugs were given over a long period.

By rational reasons, no drugs will ever be able to treat a fully developed senile dementia. Research into nootropic drugs may produce compounds that are possibly able to have more effective symptomatic actions.

Main classes of drugs presently used in clinical trials in senile dementia

Senile dementia of the Alzheimer type	Multi-infarct dementia
Nootropics Acetylcholine precursors Cholinergic compounds and cholinesterase inhibitors Compounds which increase brain glucose turnover	Nootropics Antihypertensive drugs

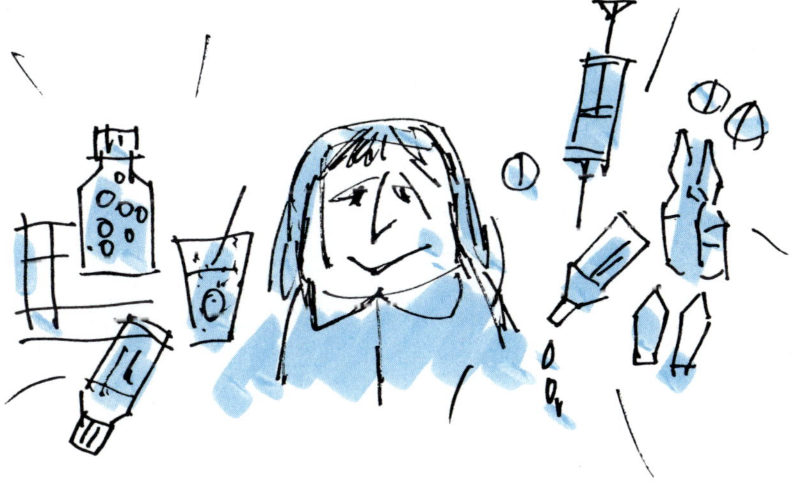

Drugs tested in Alzheimer's disease in recent years are compounds that mimic or restore the actions of brain acetylcholine.

The Value of Cerebral Vasodilators and Antihypertensives in the Treatment of Senile Dementia and Multi-Infarct Dementia

Vasodilator Drugs

These compounds relax smooth muscle in the walls of both cerebral and extracerebral blood vessels. They were first used to treat dementia. This was the time when it was thought, incorrectly, that dementia was caused by global cerebral ischaemia.

It is a fact that brain blood flow and oxygen consumption are usually below normal in patients with senile dementia of the Alzheimer type. Thus, despite the reduced brain blood flow in senile dementia of the Alzheimer type, it appears that the vascular supply is sufficient to meet the metabolic needs of the brain. Consequently drugs that increase brain blood flow have no prospect of producing any benefit as proven by numerous clinical trials.

It was suggested that vasodilators might benefit at least in multi-infarct (vascular) dementia by improving the circulation to damaged tissue, but clinical trials have failed to show any clear-cut beneficial effects of vasodilator drugs in cases of multi-infarct dementia.

Antihypertensive Drugs

The importance of treating hypertension in order to recude the risk of multi-infarct dementia is accepted. Even when a vascular dementia is apparent, antihypertensive treatment may still be useful. Not only might the risk of further infarcts be lessened, but there is evidence that hypertension per se is associated with intellectual decline in older persons. In a clinical investigation of subjects with hypertension and multi-infarct dementia, control of blood pressure to the upper limits of the normal range (135–150 mm Hg) led to improved cognition and clinical course.

Cerebral vasodilators seem to have little or no value in the treatment of either senile dementia of the Alzheimer type or in multi-infarct dementia. Reductions of arterial blood pressure in hypertensive individuals with multi-infarct dementia may be useful.

Drugs used in the treatment of locally reduced cerebral blood flow

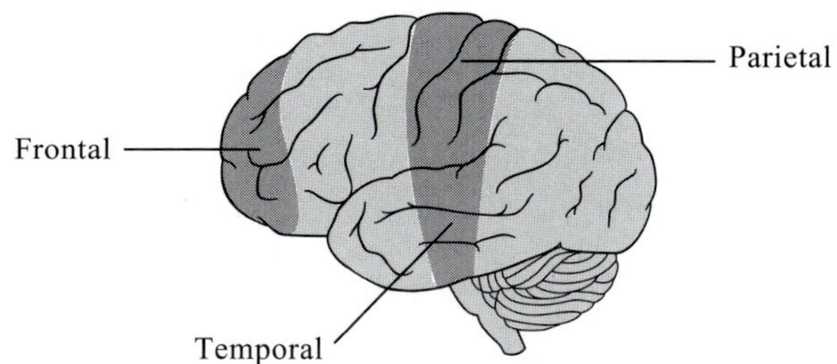

Senile dementia of the Alzheimer type is associated with cortical hypometabolism caused by a degeneration of nerve cells, which reduces the oxygen requirement of those parts of the brain most affected, which cannot be influenced by vasodilators.

Symptomatic drugs in the treatment of multi-infarct dementia: Cinnarizine (Stugeron®), co-dergocrine (Hydergine), cyclandelate, isoxsuprine, vincamine. Co-dergocrine (Hydergine) in high doses (4 mg/day or more) is considered to be effective in the treatment of multi-infarct dementia.

Caution in lowering blood pressure in multi-infarct dementia

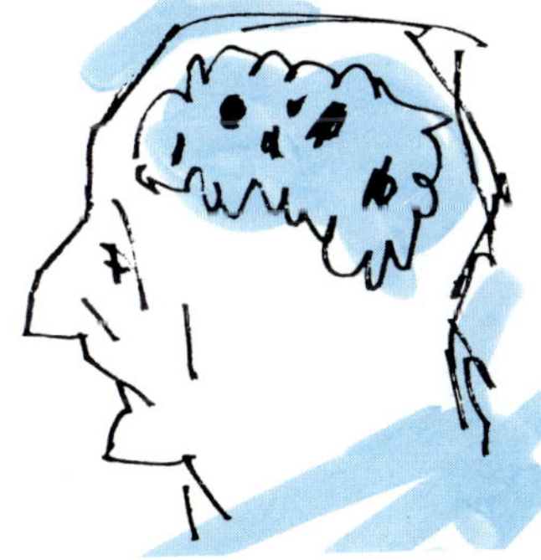

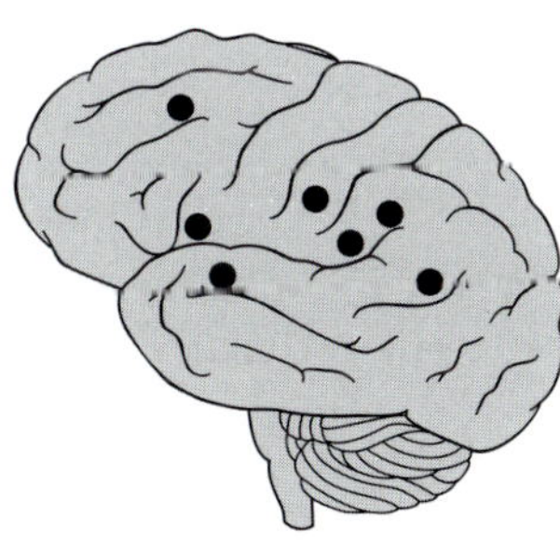

Lowering of blood pressure with antihypertensive drugs always needs to be done cautiously. Long-standing hypertension alters the threshold for autoregulation of cerebral blood vessels, such that higher-than-normal pressures are needed to maintain optimal brain perfusion.

Cholinesterase Inhibitors and Cholinergic Drugs for Treating Senile Dementia

Drugs that inhibit the enzyme cholinesterase will increase and prolong the actions of acetylcholine in the brain. Anticholinesterase treatment for senile dementia of the Alzheimer type has been tried in an attempt to overcome the decline in acetylcholine release that inevitably accompanies the degeneration of cholinergic neurons.

Physostigmine has been tested many times with some slight benefits reported, although many patients have not responded. Physostigmine has several drawbacks as a drug; it is a weak cholinesterase inhibitor with a very narrow dose range and is poorly tolerated.

Tacrine® (THA, 9-amino-1,2,3,4-tetrahydroacridine), which is a longer acting cholinesterase inhibitor, was introduced in 1986 as a long-term treatment for senile dementia. The initial report generated a lot of interest because of the benefits claimed. THA promised to be a specific treatment for senile dementia of the Alzheimer type. Long-term trials with many patients are taking place and THA has shown that serious side-effects are more pronounced than improvement of cognition.

Drugs that directly activate muscarinic receptors have been used as replacement therapy for acetylcholine in Alzheimer's disease. These include arecoline and some novel muscarinic agonists. Once again, the generally poor responses seen with these compounds may be partly explained by their limitations as effective pharmacological agents.

So far, cholinesterase inhibitors and cholinergic compounds have had only little success as therapeutic agents in senile dementia of the Alzheimer type. More potent, centrally acting compounds under development may hopefully offer better prospects.

The cholinergic synapsis in the brain as target in drug treatment of senile dementia of the Alzheimer type

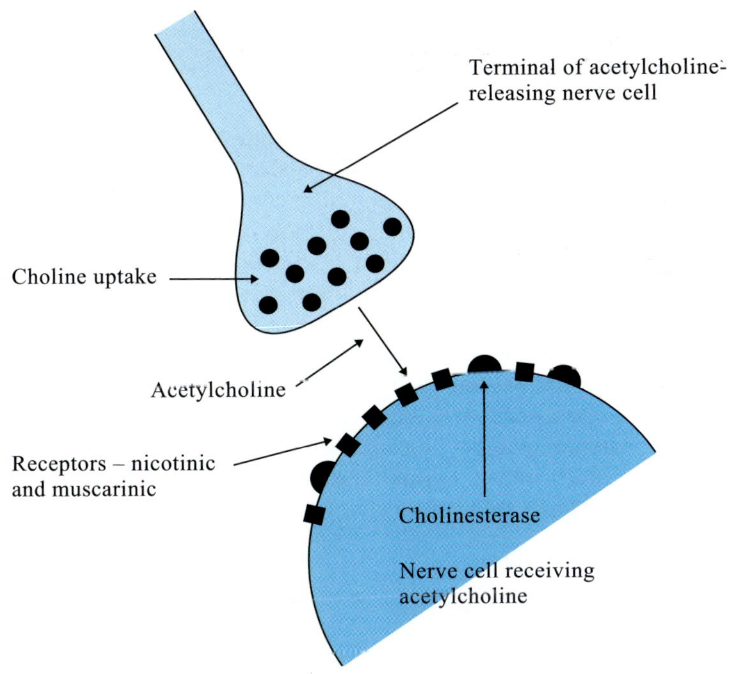

Among the drugs that have been tested in Alzheimer's disease to try to improve cognition and memory loss are compounds which may:

- either increase acetylcholine synthesis by providing a precursor (choline, lecithin),
- or inhibit cholinesterase (anticholinesterases),
- or stimulate muscarinic receptors (cholinergic compounds),
- or stimulate nicotinic receptors (nicotinic compounds).

All these approaches have up to now not been substantially successful.

What Are the Therapeutic Trends in the Treatment of Ischaemic Brain Lesions?

Compounds That Block the Actions of Glutamate
There is experimental evidence that brain glutamate released by ischaemic episodes causes damage to brain cells. Pharmacological agents that block the actions of glutamate can prevent ischaemia-induced nerve cell damage in experimental animals. If suitable compounds can be developed, glutamate blockers may be effective anti-ischaemic agents.

Calcium Channel Blockers
Calcium enters and damages brain cells made hypoxic by impairment of the blood supply. Drugs that block the specific channels for calcium in membranes of brain cells may be beneficial in conditions where perfusion of parts of the brain is reduced by vascular disease.
Drugs that block entry of calcium into cells have potent vasodilating and negative chronotropic actions and are used to treat heart disease, hypertension, and arrhythmia. Most of them have little effect on neuronal calcium channels, which are different from the channels in cardiac cells and smooth muscle. Blockers of the so-called 'L' (neuronal) calcium channels, for example nimodipine, reduce calcium entry into neurons.
However, calcium channel blockers need to be used with great caution, especially when multi-infarct dementia is suspected. A substantial fall in blood pressure could have an adverse effect on cerebral perfusion.

The development of compounds that block the neurotoxic actions of glutamate will be useful in the treatment of ischaemic brain lesions. Neuron-specific calcium channel blocking drugs represent another potential treatment for multi-infarct dementia.

The pharmacology of glutamate – a promising possibility for drug development

Nerve cells in the brain have specific receptors for the neurotransmitter glutamate. There are several types of glutamate receptors; the subtype of receptor that is most closely involved in the neurotoxic actions of glutamate is the N-methyl-*D*-aspartate-preferring receptor.

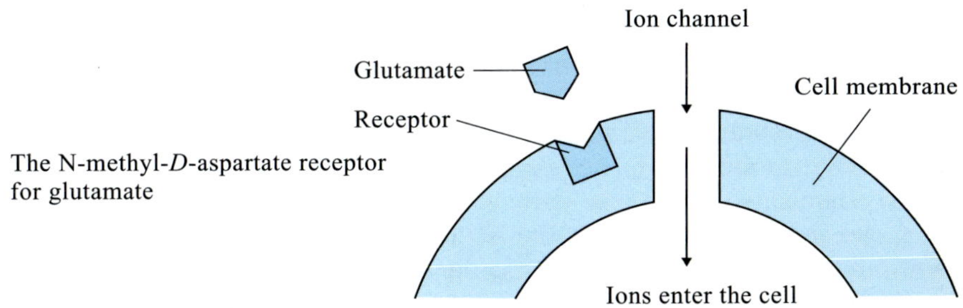

The N-methyl-*D*-aspartate receptor for glutamate

When an excess of glutamate is present it activates the receptor and opens the associated ion channel. Ions, including calcium, can enter the cells and may exert potentially damaging effects on the cell and the membrane. This is the basis of the neurotoxic action of glutamate.

Among the cells that may be damaged by overactivity of glutamate in Alzheimer's disease are the pyramidal cells in the cerebral cortex.

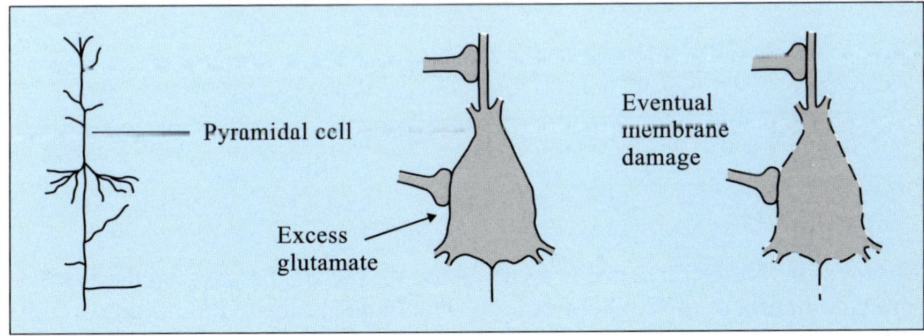

Pharmacological agents have been found which can prevent the neurotoxic action of glutamate. They include: compounds that block the N-methyl-*D*-aspartate receptor; compounds that block the membrane ion channels.

Does Nerve Growth Factor Play a Part in Senile Dementia of the Alzheimer Type?

One of the theories of Alzheimer's disease is the lack of a specific trophic factor in the brain. Nerve growth factor is important for neuronal maturation and regulation in the central and peripheral nervous systems. Nerve growth factor seems to be important not only in the developing brain but also in the mature organism.

Nerve growth factor may be linked to Alzheimer's disease because the synthesized protein messenger RNA was found in high concentrations in neurons in the cerebral cortex and hippocampus, brain areas that show extensive neurodegeneration in Alzheimer's disease. Equally significant is that messenger RNA for the nerve growth factor receptor is most abundant in the septum and basal forebrain where the cholinergic neurons that project to hippocampus and cortex are found. Nerve growth factor and its receptors are therefore closely associated with those parts of the brain that show the most serious damages in senile dementia of the Alzheimer type.

An important question is whether senile dementia involves the failure of an essential supply of nerve growth factor from target cortical and hippocampal neurons. The answer to this question is not known, but treatment based on nerve growth factor might be used, one day, to slow the neurodegeneration of cholinergic neurons in senile dementia of the Alzheimer type. Encouraging results were obtained with experimental animals where nerve growth factor prevented cholinergic neuron degeneration produced by a neurotoxic substance related to glutamate.

Absence or failure of nerve growth factor is one of the suggested causes of senile dementia of the Alzheimer type. The factor is needed to maintain some of the nerve cells that degenerate in senile dementia and can prevent degeneration of acetylcholine nerve cells in experimental animals. There are as yet no treatments available which can be used to replace this trophic factor in man.

Do brain cells degenerate in senile dementia of the Alzheimer type because they lack a trophic factor?

One trophic factor that has been identified in the brain is the nerve growth factor. This not only helps immature nerve cells to develop, but also maintains adult brain cells.

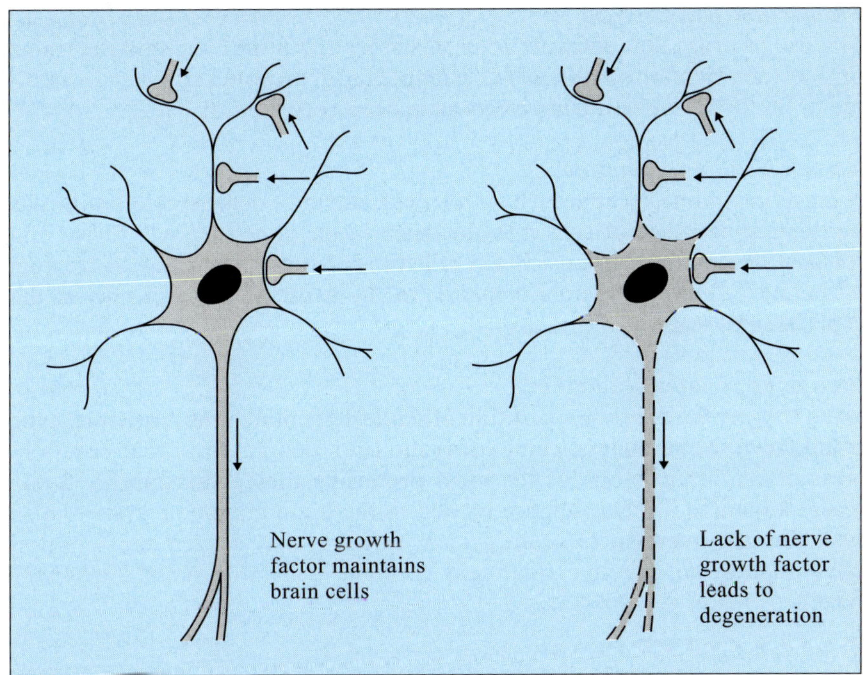

The experimental findings with nerve growth factor cannot yet be exploited for the treatment of senile dementia of the Alzheimer type. A major problem for therapy is poor passage of nerve growth factor across the blood-brain barrier, and major advances in drug delivery systems will be needed before either nerve growth factor or compounds with similar pharmacological actions can be used therapeutically.

How Great Is the Chance to Develop an Effective Treatment for Senile Dementia of the Alzheimer Type?

The major obstacle to be overcome in designing treatments for senile dementia is that it is a degenerative condition in which brain cells in some parts of the brain are progressively destroyed. In common with other neurodegenerative conditions, senile dementia of the Alzheimer type is proving to be highly resistant to treatment.

Transmitter Replacement
The use of drugs that activate brain receptors and mimic the missing transmitters (acetylcholine is the prime example) is an accepted strategy for treatment. So far the benefits described have been very modest.

Nerve Cell Transplantation
A far more ambitious approach is the replacement of degenerated brain cells by implanting tissue or cells into the brain in the hope they will thrive and replace the missing neurons. Brain cell transplantation as a way of treating Alzheimer's disease or senile dementia of the Alzheimer type is only at the experimental stage.

Preventing Neurodegeneration
What triggers the neurodegeneration of senile dementia of the Alzheimer type is unknown. Nevertheless, combatting the neurodegeneration that occurs in parts of the brain is one of the most promising therapeutic targets. Some recent advances in neuroscience related to the brain glutamate system, or a systemic improvement of brain glucose turnover and oxygen consumption offer hope of an effective treatment of senile dementia of the Alzheimer type.

Several prospective treatments for degenerative disorders, including senile dementia of the Alzheimer type, are at the experimental stage.

The transplantation approach for transmitter replacement in senile dementia

Several attempts have been made in recent years to compensate for the degeneration of brain dopamine neurons that is the hallmark of Parkinson's disease by transplanting dopamine-producing cells from a fetus into the key brain areas of Parkinson's disease victims. Although this type of surgical approach to the treatment of neurodegenerative diseases is very much in its infancy, it has been suggested that Alzheimer's disease might, one day, be treated by grafting tissue or transplanting cholinergic neurons into the brain.

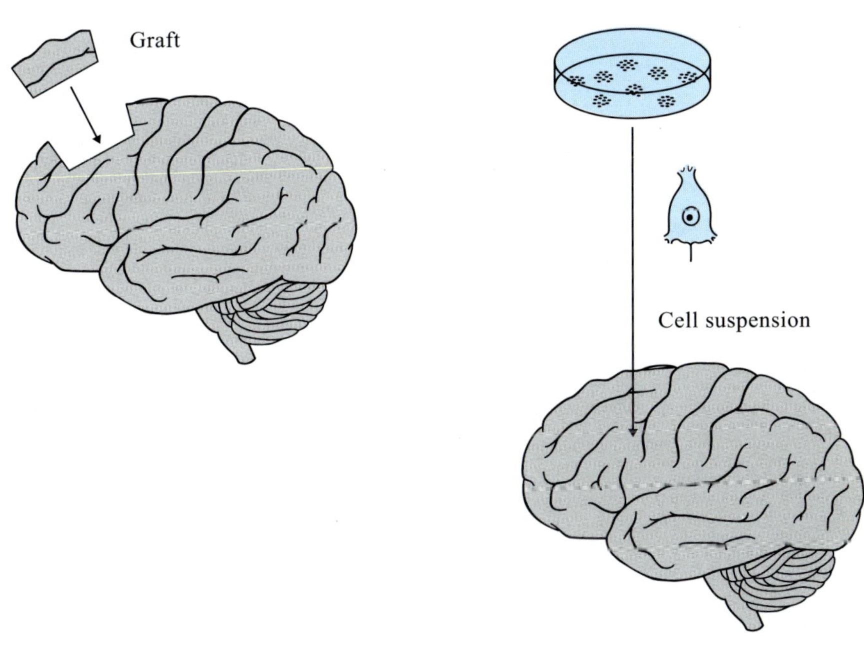

Work on experimental animals has shown that fetal acetylcholine neurons, in the form of grafts or cell suspensions, transplanted into the brain will survive, grow and make some functional connections with other cells. The difficulties in applying this type of approach to senile dementia of the Alzheimer type are: the widespread neurodegeneration involving several parts of the brain, and the fact that several important transmitters, not just acetylcholine, disappear from the brain.

Coping with Senile Dementia

B. Forette

Accurate Differential Diagnosis – An Expensive Business

Various diseases may simulate senile dementia or presenile dementia. Some of these can be treated, so that if a patient presents with signs of dementia, it is important to assemble all the data needed for differential diagnosis.

The number of people with dementia in the population is large (about 5%), but only a limited number of these can be treated. The cost of the investigations involved in a systematic search for a curable cause of dementia may appear to be high, but the costs of long-term treatment and of institutional care are significantly higher.

Once Alzheimer's disease or vascular dementia has been diagnosed, the family can be properly advised. The patient should be spared treatments which are of no value. Periodic evaluation of the stages of the disorder is a help in determining the general course of action and predicting as early as possible what measures are likely to be necessary in the future. The choice of institution can also be made well in advance and under favourable circumstances.

Although dementia rarely has a cause which is amenable to treatment, a systemic search for such a cause is justified. The investigations are not unduly expensive, considering the advantages they offer. Accurate diagnosis and periodic evaluation make it possible to select in good time those aids likely to be of greatest value.

Curable causes of a dementia syndrome must be identified as early as possible

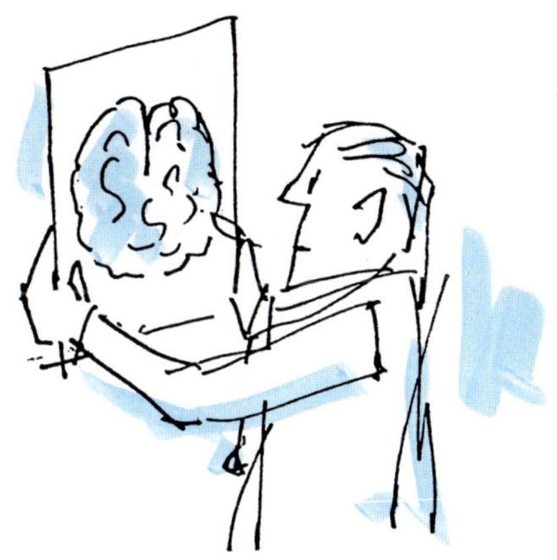

A diagnosis of irreversible dementia has serious implications. Before giving the family, and sometimes the patient, such a grave prognosis, it is wise to eliminate possible causes which are amenable to treatment. Special methods of investigation are needed.

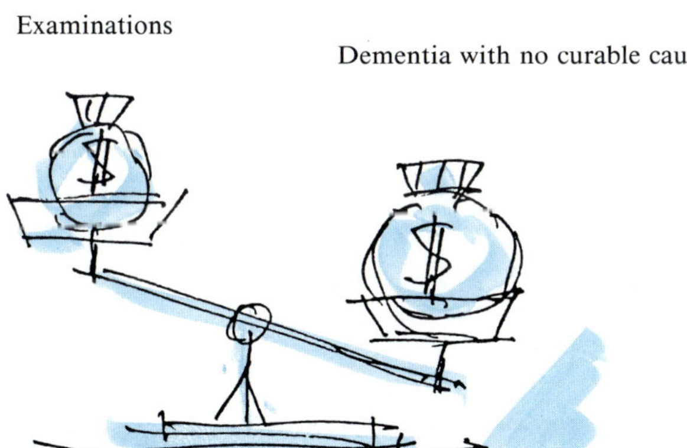

The search for a curable cause of dementia in every patient is a costly undertaking and will identify only a small number of treatable cases.

Dementia Is Always a Disease with a Protracted Course

The time that will elapse between the first occurrence of the symptoms and the death of the patient cannot be exactly predicted. A study published in 1985 indicated a mean course of 8.5 years for Alzheimer's disease. For dementia of vascular origin the mean course was reported to be 6.7 years. The cause of death is usually an intercurrent disease.

If patients survive long enough they eventually become completely helpless. The burden imposed on those caring for the patient changes as time passes. Coming to terms with changes in behaviour and personality is thought to be the most difficult problem for some. As the dementia progresses and the patient becomes weaker, less mobile and progressively aphasic, behavioural disorders might be thought to be less of a problem. In actual fact it is generally agreed that the burden on those caring for the patient increases steadily as the dementia progressively worsens. The cost of care to the family and to society follows the same pattern.

About 5 out of 6 patients with dementia are looked after at home, but the proportion declines significantly when the disease reaches an advanced stage. Seven out of 10 patients attending a day hospital either died or were admitted to an institution within 1 year. Whether a patient is cared for at home depends more on how supportive the family is than on the state of the patient.

Dementia usually develops over a number of years. Most patients live at home, but as time goes on more and more of them are admitted to institutions. Whether a patient is admitted to an institution depends more on how supportive the family is than on the state of the patient.

The critical question: home care or nursing home?

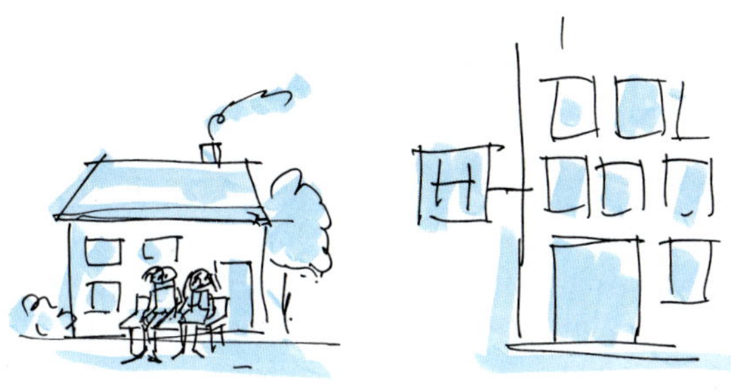

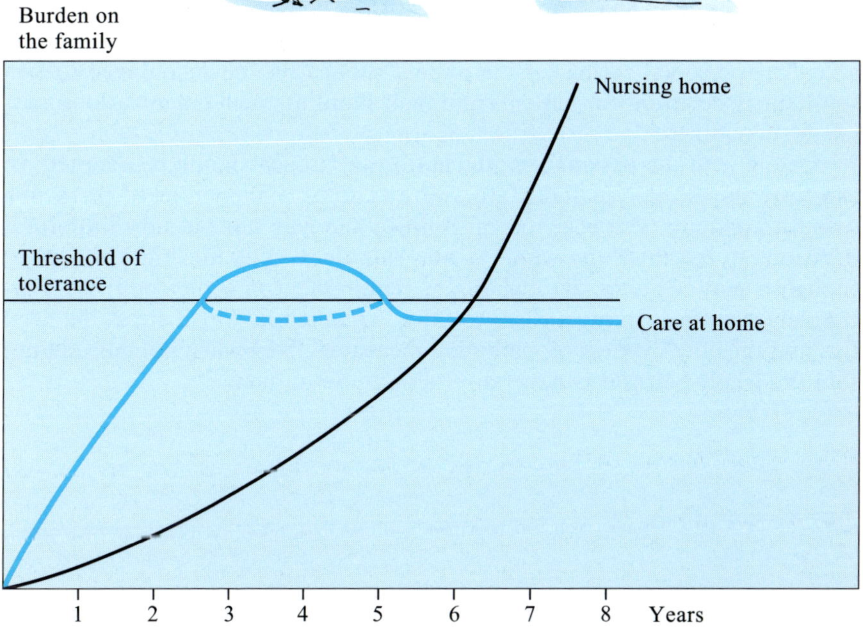

Burden on the family

Nursing home

Threshold of tolerance

Care at home

1 2 3 4 5 6 7 8 Years

In most cases the burden becomes progressively more onerous as the patient's condition deteriorates (black curve). In other cases (blue curve) behavioural disturbances are the biggest problem and push the burden on the family beyond the threshold of physical and psychological tolerance, causing admission to an institution. Those caring for the patient would be able to 'survive' the critical period if massive aid was provided to ensure that the threshold of tolerance was not exceeded (broken line) while the disease followed its natural course.

What Should the Patient and the Immediate Family Be Told in Cases of a Dementing Brain Disease?

It is preferable to inform those close to the patient as soon as the diagnosis of dementia syndrome is reasonably certain, in order to give the family time to take steps to cope. The raising of false hopes must be avoided because it damages the doctor's credibility and poisons future relations. Honesty is not incompatible with a tactful approach towards less resilient people, to whom the facts should be unfolded gradually. Several counselling sessions will nearly always be necessary. The information imparted must be presented in a form comprehensible to the person(s) concerned. The doctor must not be frightened of repeating himself, many times if necessary. It is worth verifying that the most important messages have been properly understood and correctly interpreted. The family must feel that it is receiving the support it needs and emphasis must be placed on the various forms of assistance available. The person(s) caring for the patient should also be encouraged to join self-help associations for patients and their families. Such organizations exist in most countries.

In dealing with the patient a more cautious approach should be adopted. In the early stages many patients are aware of what is happening to them. We owe it to patients who bear responsibilities and who have to take important decisions to tell them the whole truth. This right to be told the truth, hard though it may be, is in fact a statutory requirement in some countries. Fortunately it suffices in most cases to offer explanations which stress the need for, and the effectiveness of, palliative measures. Even when patients are not told the whole truth, it is never advisable to lie to them.

Right from the onset of Alzheimer's disease those caring for the patient must be informed about the course the disease will take. What patients are told depends upon the circumstances and the particular case. It is never advisable to tell them downright lies.

The truth about the course and outcome of Alzheimer's disease is painful but unavoidable

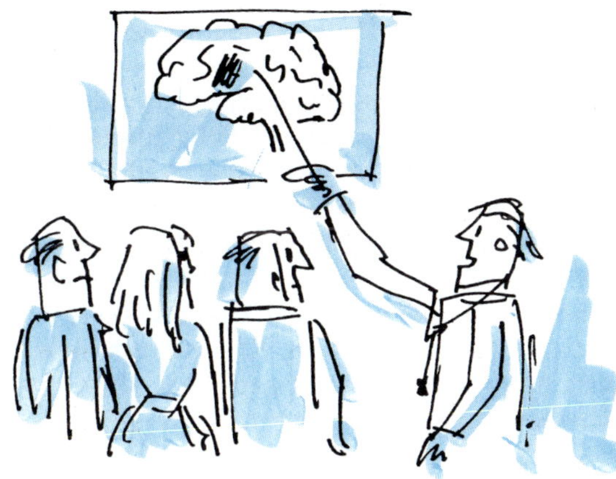

The information given must be honest, as complete as possible and capable of being understood by the family.

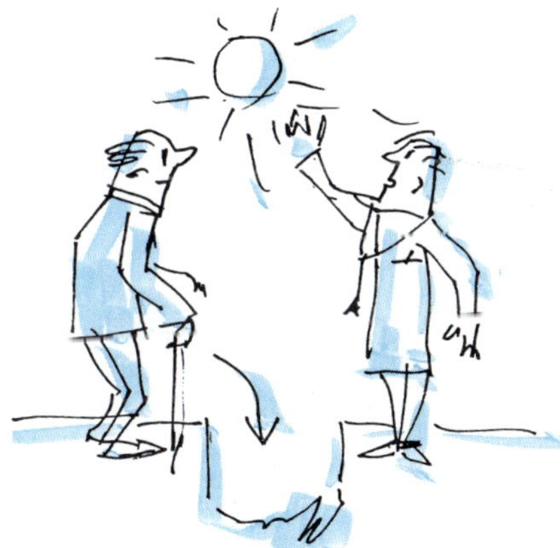

Some patients have to know the whole truth as early as possible. Others may be given more sketchy information, with the accent on palliative measures. Telling deliberate lies must be avoided.

Recognition and Treatment of Intercurrent Diseases in the Course of a Dementing Brain Disease

In elderly persons polypathia is common, but in demented individuals concomitant diseases frequently go unrecognized because dementia masks or distorts other signs of disease. Patients either do not complain or their complaints are inappropriate. Patients' responses to questioning cannot be relied upon, even when they are able to express themselves. The patient must therefore be thoroughly examined for latent disorders at every consultation.
Somatic disorders affect behaviour, often misinterpreted as an exacerbation of the dementia. Pain, fever, and metabolic disorders frequently induce agitation or aggressiveness. Dehydration, anaemia, heart failure and numerous drug-induced side-effects may aggravate cognitive disorders.
Any unusual sign should prompt a search for a disease associated with the dementia. Thorough clinical examination is mandatory, but clinical findings alone are often not enough. Extensive use must be made of special investigations, imaging techniques and laboratory tests. Disorders which most frequently go unrecognized are:

- fractures, especially of the limbs, femoral neck, pelvis, ribs and vertebrae,
- retention of urine,
- otitis and stomatitis,
- chronic haemorrhage leading to iron deficiency anaemia;
- chronic ulcers etc.

In dementia intercurrent diseases are often missed. Patients must be thoroughly examined at regular intervals, particularly when dementia appears to be worsening without good reason. Treatment of these concomitant disorders may greatly improve the patient's behaviour.

The worsening of a dementia syndrome is often the result of a somatic disease

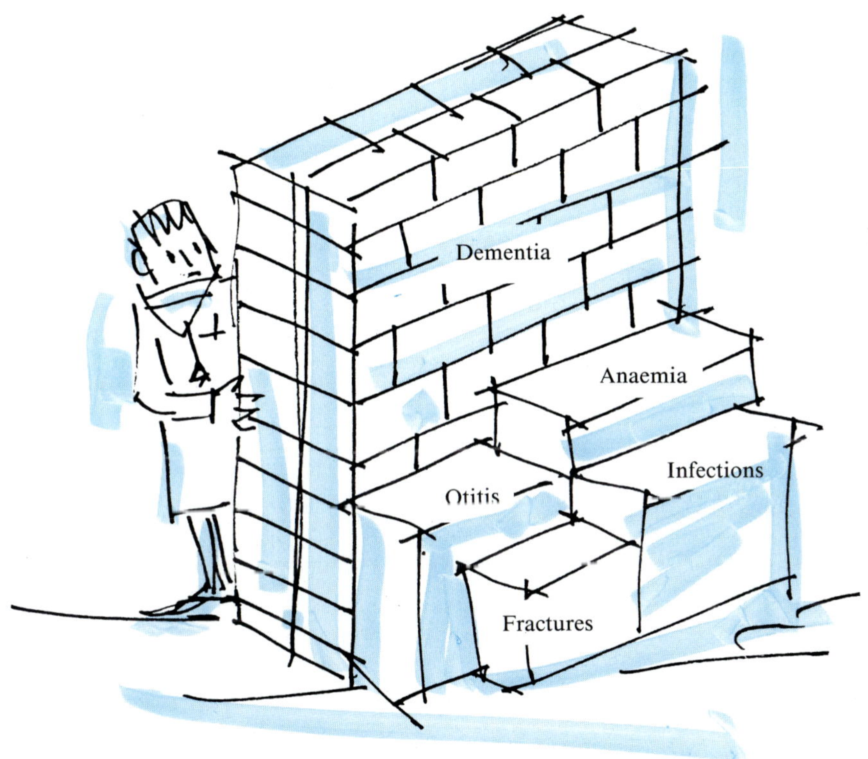

Dementia frequently masks other disorders. These are only discovered if they are sought as a matter of course.

Polypharmacy or as Few Drugs as Possible?

Prescription of drugs is a delicate matter affecting relations between the doctor and those caring for the patient. Conscientious, overprotective persons expect the doctor to prescribe medication for every sign or symptom. The family must be given to understand that it is not possible to relieve each and every symptom. A priority list must be drawn up and some symptoms accepted in view of the seriousness of therapeutic accidents. A less caring family may think that if a large number of drugs are administered, this makes up for their failure to look after the patient better.

Patients themselves are often very attached to drugs of dubious value. They may also refuse to take drugs which they really need. Lengthy explanations, a great deal of time and much patience are needed to gain acceptance for a reasonable therapeutic regimen.

Several chronic disorders frequently coexist in senile dementia. Each requires one, and often several, forms of long-term therapy. The situation may easily get out of hand, leading to unpredictable drug interactions.

At each consultation the whole medication regimen should be carefully reviewed. This rule does not apply merely to drugs prescribed for the patient's comfort, such as analgesics and hypnotics. Major 'life-line treatments' such as digitalis, antihypertensive agents, oral hypoglycaemic agents etc. should be reviewed. Are they still indicated? Can the dosage be reduced? Do the advantages outweigh the drawbacks?

A number of factors are conducive to the potentially dangerous escalation of drug ingestion in elderly patients with dementia. It is a question of knowing how to limit the number of drugs prescribed, rather than trying to treat everything.

The demented patient is always suffering from numerous other acute or chronic disorders

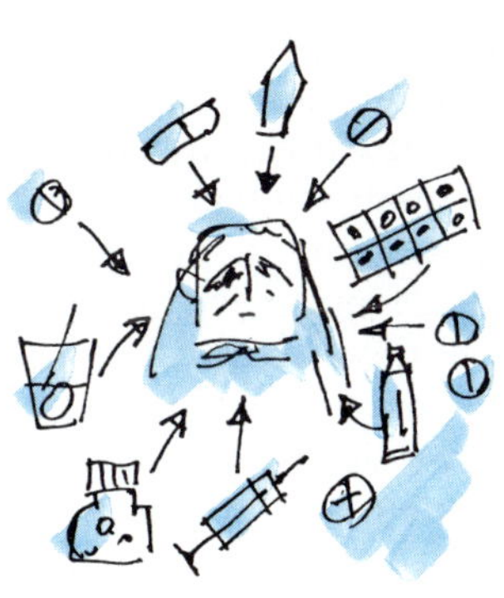

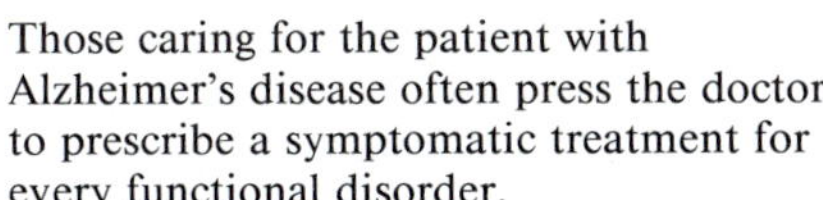

Those caring for the patient with Alzheimer's disease often press the doctor to prescribe a symptomatic treatment for every functional disorder.

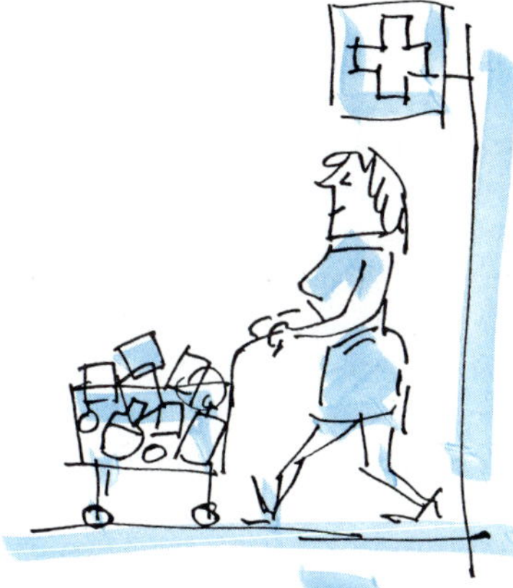

Many drugs are purchased over the counter. Consumption of drugs soon becomes excessive.

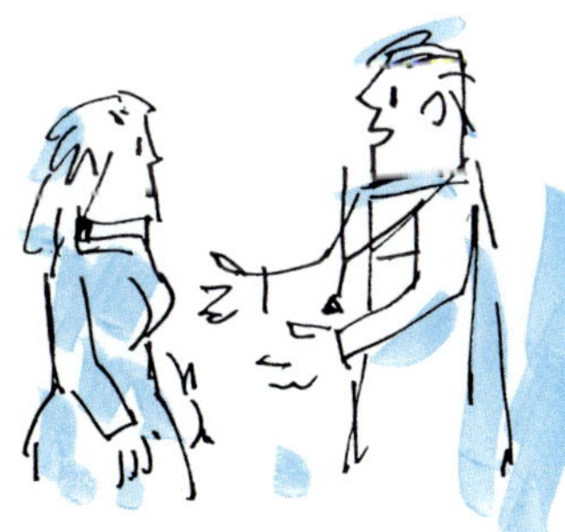

It takes time and patience to convince families that it is not desirable to treat each and every sign and symptom.

The Risk of Side-Effects

Like all elderly people, patients with dementia take many drugs of all kinds, but in dementia drug side-effects are probably more frequent and harder to recognize.
Many drugs may affect cognitive functions, induce agitation or confusional states. There is a real danger that these signs and symptoms may be attributed to exacerbation of the dementia. This is particularly important with psychotropic drugs, i.e. hypnotics, tranquillizers, antipsychotic drugs, anticonvulsants and antidepressants. A common error is to increase the dosage or to add another psychotropic drug instead of discontinuing the drug in question or reducing the dosage. Many other classes of drugs may be implicated in inducing serious side-effects, e.g. digitalis derivatives, antihypertensive agents, cimetidine, theophylline, oral hypoglycaemic agents, anticholinergics, diuretics, etc. Patients have frequently been taking these drugs for a long time without apparent adverse effects. Often toxic effects are noticed when a drug interaction occurs with another new treatment.
Conversely, dementia may mask or lessen the symptoms of a drug side-effect. Also, patients are frequently incapable of drawing attention to the symptoms they are experiencing. The danger is that intoxication will pass unrecognized until more serious complications supervene. Signs of drug intolerance must be looked for systematically at routine consultations. Where there is any doubt, the doctor should have no hesitation in requesting laboratory tests or drug plasma level assays.

Drug side-effects are even more common in patients with dementia than in other geriatric patients. The possibility of drug side-effects should always be borne in mind whenever dementia suddenly worsens. Signs of drug intoxication should be looked for systematically at each routine consultation.

Demented patients are more vulnerable than others to drug intoxication

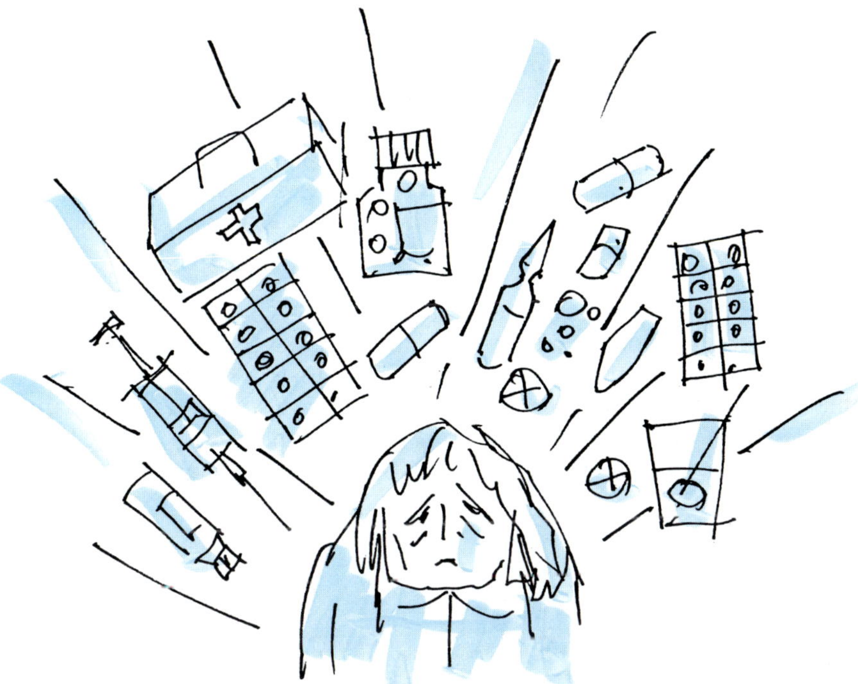

The increased vulnerability of demented patients to drug side-effects results from the fact:

- that they take more drugs,
- that they are more sensitive to certain side-effects, and
- that signs of intoxication are harder to recognize in such patients.

Agitation, an Important Alarm Symptom in Alzheimer Patients

Agitation, hyperactivity and aggressiveness are sometimes simply due to the fact that the patient has lost the ability to express himself properly. Hyperactivity and aggressiveness are his way of indicating that he is experiencing discomfort (excessively tight clothing), pain (injury, burns, joint pain, neuralgia, toothache), illness (fever, an infection), or anxiety (departure of a person close to the patient, change of environment). If no obvious reason can be found in the patient's environment he should be examined clinically to discover possible somatic causes.

Agitation may also result from drug intolerance. If the doctor, instead of exploring the reason for the patient's agitation, simply prescribes a sedative, he risks adding a second intoxication to the first. Paradoxical reactions (e.g. to benzodiazepines) are more common in the elderly.

Regular physical exercise during the day reduces the risk of agitation. If patients engage in sporting activities, they should be advised to continue to do so for as long as they are able.

If neuroleptic treatment has to be given, then certain rules should be observed: The doctor should choose the drug with which he is most familiar. In particular, he should only prescribe one drug at a time. Thioridazine and haloperidol are the most frequently prescribed drugs. Treatment is started at one third or one half of the adult dosage, progressively increasing until the minimum effective level is attained. If the patient develops symptoms of parkinsonism with haloperidol, the therapy may be changed to thioridazine.

If a patient becomes agitated, the first task is to discover the cause: it could be a side-effect of a drug, a change in the environment, an injury, pain or an intercurrent disease.

The inability of the senile demented patient to express himself is compensated for by agitation

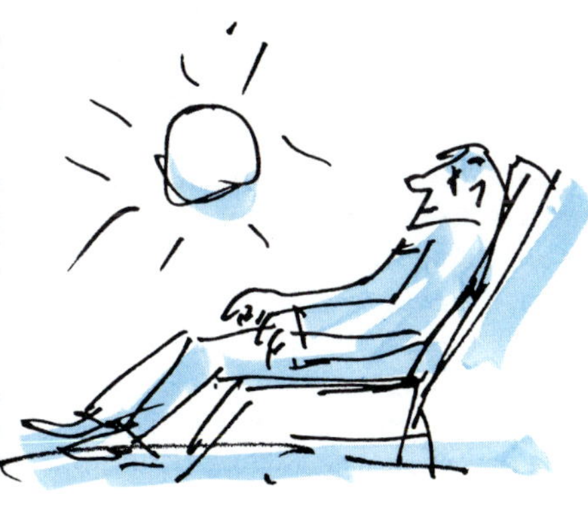

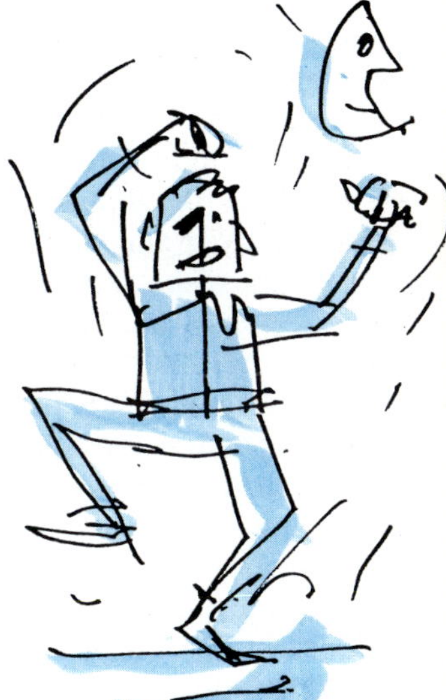

Inactivity during the day predisposes to nocturnal agitation.

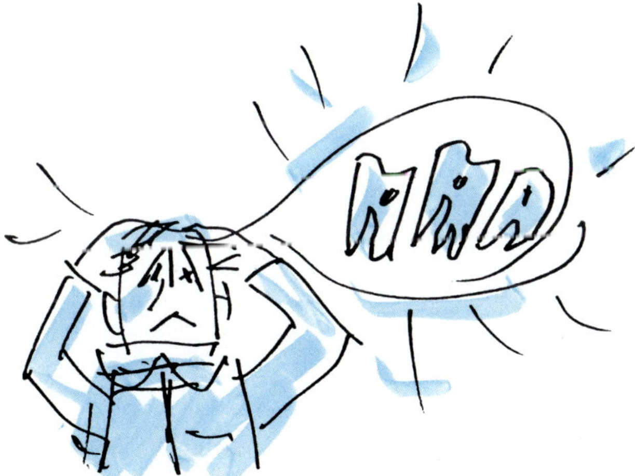

Agitation is sometimes a manifestation of physical pain or discomfort which the patient cannot express in other ways.

Insomnia in the Demented Patient, a Serious Burden for Nursing Staff and the Family

Insomnia in demented patients affects those looking after them, for they too need a good night's sleep. Insomnia is frequently accompanied by nocturnal wandering and inappropriate behaviour. The patient may dress, have breakfast and go out in the middle of the night. In dementia the sleep-wake cycle is disrupted by the disease itself, but often external factors may be involved. Lack of activity and lack of work during the day are not conducive to sleeping through the night. A long walk at the end of the afternoon sometimes normalizes sleeping habits. Mentally stimulating activities may be substituted for the afternoon rest. A comfortable bed, a congenial bedroom temperature and a stable environment are important prerequisites, but the patient is not capable of voicing complaints when things are not what they should be. By attending to these factors it may be possible to avoid giving hypnotics. Adherence to an unchanging bedtime ritual may induce sleep. Some patients find a nightlight helps them sleep, others find it a hindrance to sleeping.

However, hypnotics may sometimes prove indispensable, in particular if those caring for the patient are completely exhausted. There is no ideal hypnotic. High doses and drugs that are eliminated slowly should be avoided. A low dose of a hypnotic with a short biological half-life should be prescribed. The need for hypnotics should be reviewed frequently and even more stringently than the need for other drugs.

Insomnia in dementia may prove exhausting to those looking after the patient. Before prescribing hypnotics, negative factors should if possible be corrected, i.e. irregular habits, lack of physical activity, sleeping during the day and uncongenial bedroom conditions.

Hypnotics are the easiest but worst way of compensating for sleep disturbances in a patient with senile dementia

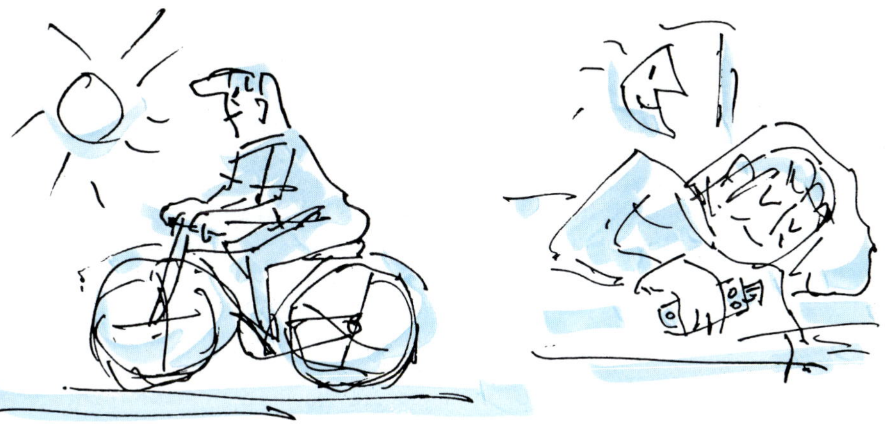

Adequate physical activity during the day, especially in the late afternoon, is conducive to a good night's sleep.

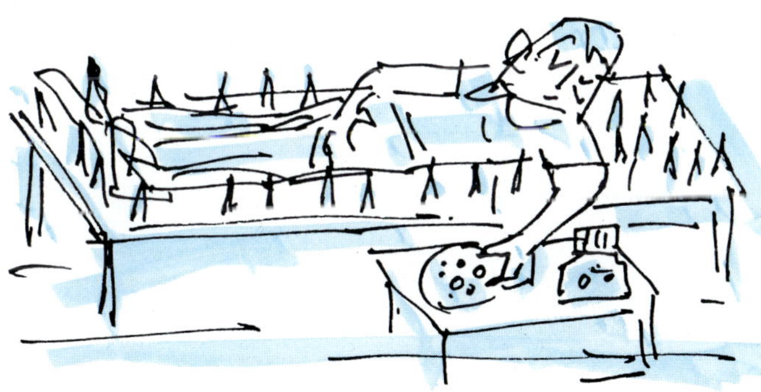

Insomnia sometimes results from an uncomfortable bedroom, which the patient is unable to complain about. A change in bedding, avoidance of noise and a pleasant bedroom temperature will avoid the need for hypnotics.

Depression – A Frequent Intercurrent Disease in Senile Dementia

Dementia is not curable, but a depressive syndrome accompanying it should be treated. These patients probably suffer as much as non-demented depressive individuals. Diagnosis is more difficult against the background of a dementia syndrome. A striking change in mood will not, however, escape the family. But the way in which the depression manifests itself may be quite atypical when verbal communication is impaired.

Depression should be suspected if the patient displays abrupt changes in behaviour, shows apathy or aggressiveness, or makes hypochondriac demands. There is a real risk of suicide. If the patient talks about dying, it is unwise to count upon it that impaired coordination or loss of memory will prevent the patient from putting words into deeds.

Among the antidepressants the tricyclic compounds are still the drugs of choice. Otherwise there are a number of drugs that may be tried such as fluvoxamine (acts on the serotonergic receptors), mianserin (has a sedative effect which is useful in sleep disturbances) or one of the new monoamine oxidase inhibitors (which have far fewer drawbacks than their predecessors).

Antidepressives must be started at a low dosage, then gradually increased. They do not act instantly, and severe depression may threaten the life of the patient in the early days. Antidepressants have many contra-indications and produce appreciable side-effects. That is why electroshock therapy is sometimes worth considering. It is a simple and effective treatment which acts rapidly and is of proven safety. It should not be brushed aside because of the irrational arguments sometimes raised against it.

Depression is common in dementia but is sometimes atypical and difficult to recognize. Depression exacerbates the disturbances due to dementia and may lead to suicide. It is normally treated with tricyclic antidepressants.

Depression in an Alzheimer patient must be treated

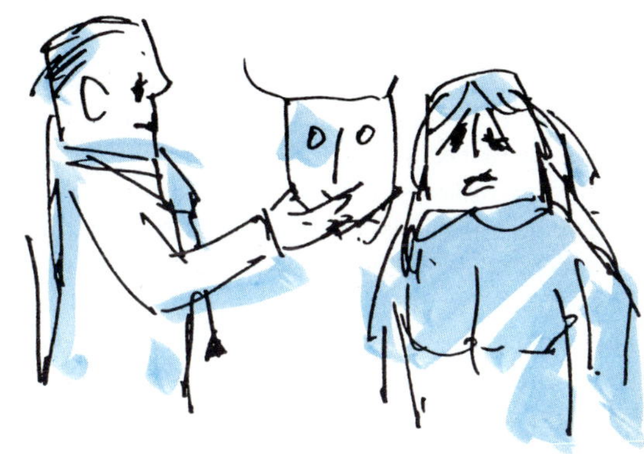

Depression may wear a deceptive mask in dementia. It is a diagnosis which should always be borne in mind when the patient's behaviour changes.

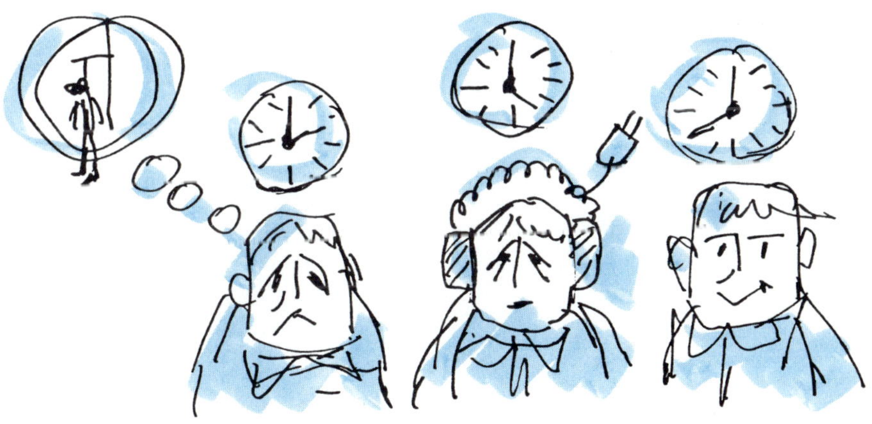

In urgent cases electroshock therapy may save the life of a patient with suicidal tendencies. It takes effect rapidly, has few contra-indications and is generally very well tolerated.

The Programmed Conflict Situation: The Family Doctor and the Others Involved

One of the most difficult of the family doctor's tasks is to co-ordinate the roles of all those involved, namely:
- the patient himself;
- the family, and more particularly the person caring for the patient;
- medical auxiliaries, nurses, helpers, physiotherapists, speech therapists, etc.;
- social workers;
- bodies providing non-medical aid;
- the hospital and various institutions;
- medical specialists.

Differences of opinion are bound to arise in this complex set-up. Some of those concerned tend to exceed their authority. Others take their responsibilities too lightly. The family doctor is expected to discharge his task as arbiter with due tact. A good way of avoiding clashes is to carefully define from the outset the extent and limits of the duties of each of those involved, taking into account their personality, abilities and scope for action.
Sometimes the family doctor may find himself in disagreement with one or several members of the team. If this happens, one overriding precept should guide his conduct: to represent the patient and defend his interests, regardless of all other considerations.

It is the job of the family doctor to co-ordinate the various people involved with the patient and to arbitrate between them when difficulties arise.

The family doctor treating the demented patient has to defend his patient's interests

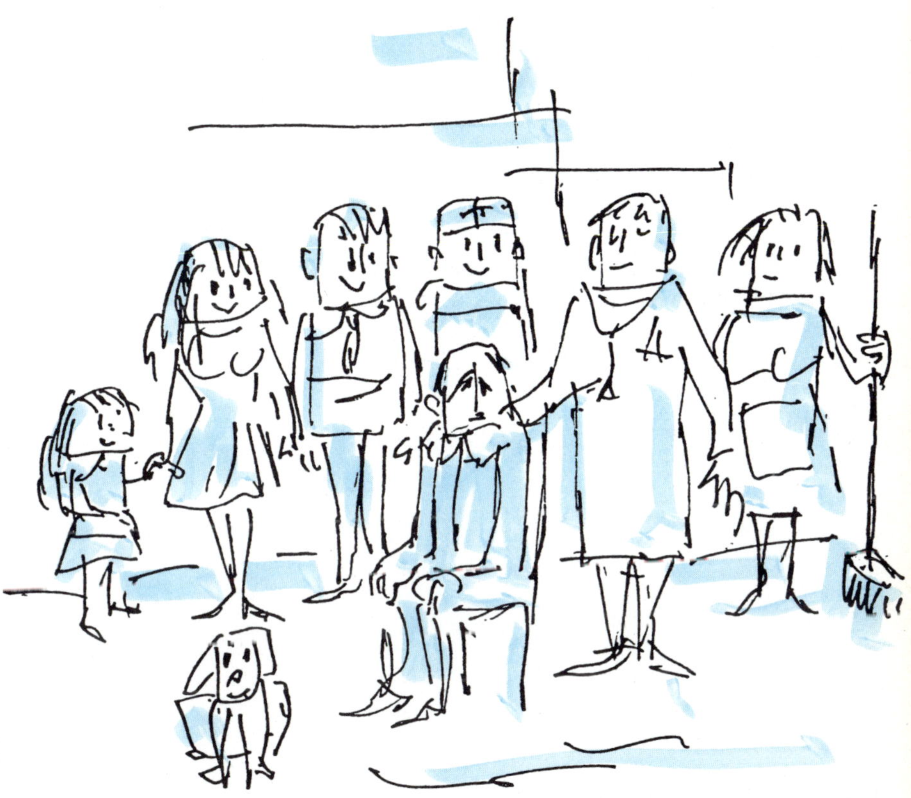

The family doctor is the natural mediator and co-ordinator for the people and organizations involved with the patient. This means that he must arbitrate in the differences which inevitably arise. He is best placed to protect the patient's interests in all circumstances.

The Role of the Family in Caring for an Alzheimer Patient

The great majority of elderly demented patients are looked after at home either by their spouse or by one of their children. The spouse is generally an elderly person, who is also suffering from various infirmities or chronic diseases and leaving the couple in their own home is a precarious equilibrium which some, on the face of it, minor incident may abruptly upset. Contingency provisions should therefore be made from the start for possible breakdown. Sometimes feelings of guilt prevent the spouse from contemplating the idea of separation, and it should be made clear that contingency planning for future options is in no way binding.

The child caring for a patient will generally be a middle-aged woman. She herself sometimes has grown-up children and her own home to look after. In other instances an unmarried daughter may have sacrificed her career. An American study indicated that 3 out of 4 persons caring for an elderly demented patient lived with the patient 7 days a week. Less than 10% took advantage of the help provided by the various organizations. The role of the family doctor is also to care for the 'carers', lending moral support and helping them to obtain all the assistance needed.

Caring for an elderly demented patient is a highly exhausting task in all respects, whoever the person on whom the responsibility falls. It is vital that the family doctor should support the 'carers'. With them he should draw up a contingency plan well in advance offering the best solution in the event that they should one day no longer be able to cope.

Caring for a patient with senile dementia is a heavy burden

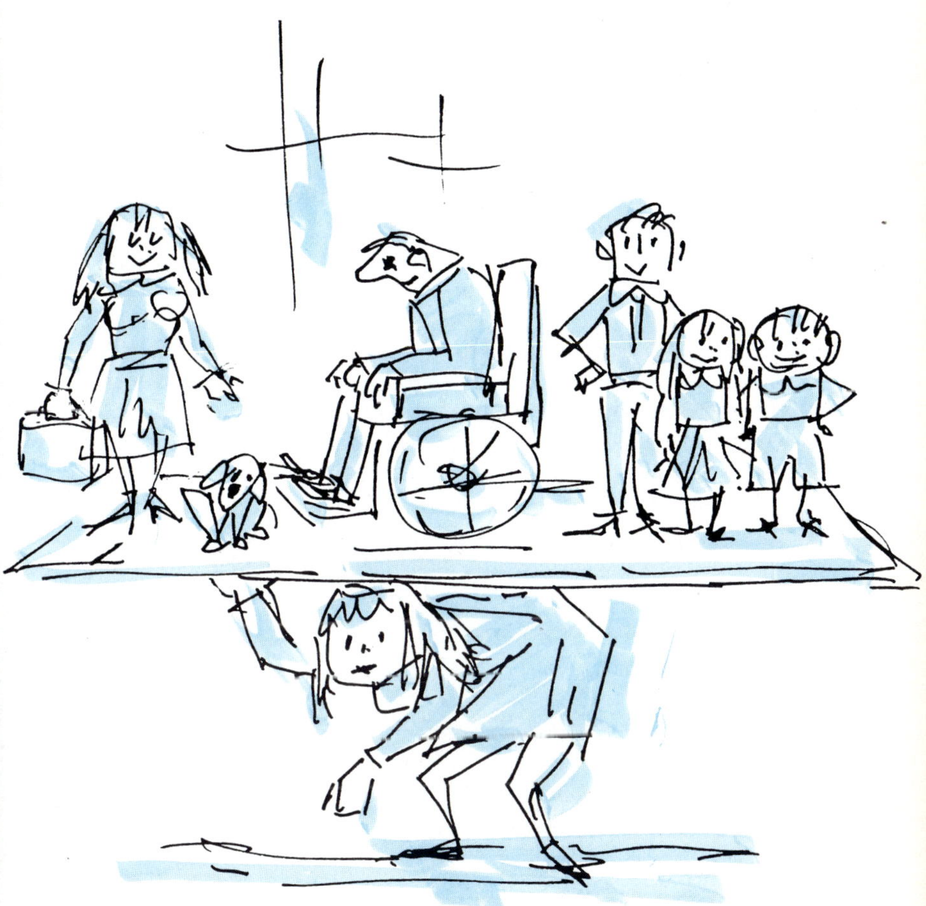

In the traditional family the demented old person was cared for by one of his or her daughters, a spinster, who had forgone a career or profession. Nowadays such people are usually married, 50 years of age or more and have a family of their own.

Help in Caring for the Patient with Senile Dementia in the Family

The provisions for home help vary greatly from country to country, region to region, one city to another, and even from one part of a city to another. Not only do the services provided differ, but also the organizations providing them, the cost and mode of financing. Patients' families usually have to apply to the local social security department to ascertain what forms of aid are available in their community, what the financial conditions are and what formalities have to be completed. More and more private organizations are coming into existence, some charitable, some profit-oriented. The help offered is of three types:

– *Nursing care* is provided either by free-lance professionals whose fees are paid by the patient's health insurance, or by services run directly by the state. Other paramedical disciplines may be involved: physiotherapists, chiropodists, speech therapists etc. These services are generally available on prescription.

– *Help with daily living activities.* Home helps carry out routine domestic tasks, do the shopping and sometimes take the patient out. Some communities provide 'meals on wheels' and laundry services. Having someone to look after the patient during the day, and especially during the night, is greatly appreciated by families, but this is also the hardest to get.

– *Help with domestic appliances* is sometimes provided for the patient's comfort and safety, e.g. removal or replacement of dangerous appliances, improvements to the heating system, etc. Alarm systems and closed-circuit television surveillance systems are sometimes maintained in whole or in part by the social security organizations.

Various forms of assistance, both private and public, ensure that the patient can be cared for at home. Generally families obtain advice on the services available from the social services department of the local authorities.

Public and private services can ease the burden on the Alzheimer patient's principal care provider

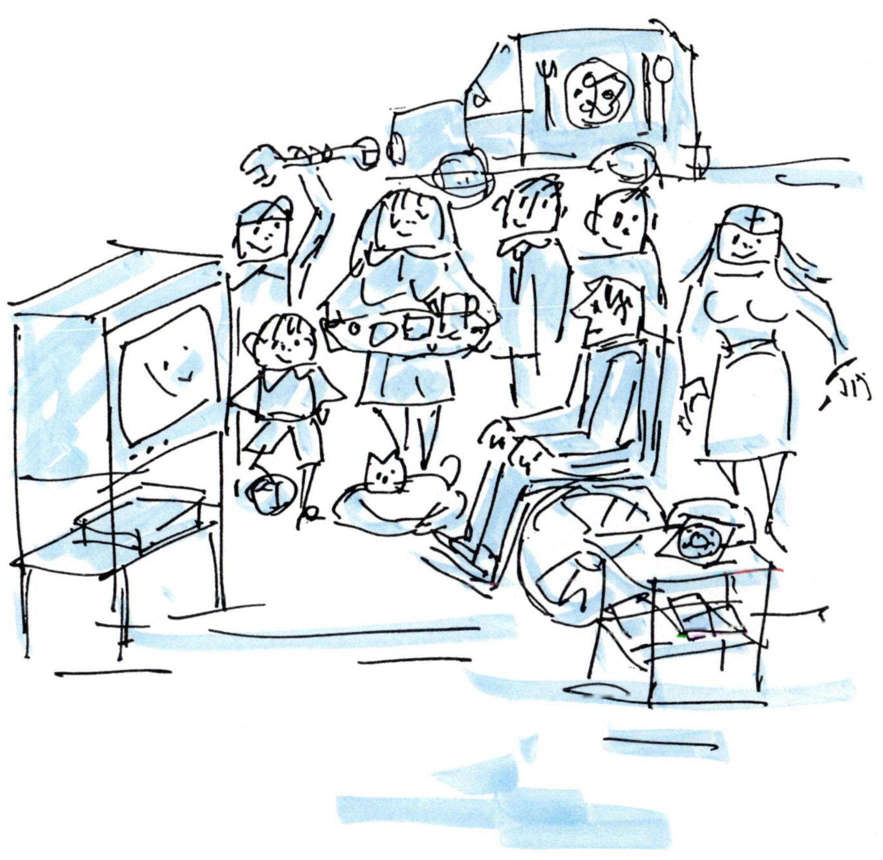

Home help services can appreciably lighten the burden on the person caring for the patient. They are a way of avoiding or deferring placement in an institution. Frequently, however, families are poorly informed about the services available.

Day Hospital and Day Centre, an Opportunity to Support the Family of a Patient with Senile Dementia

The day hospital offers most of the facilities of an ordinary hospital, but the patient returns home at night. A day hospital offers many different services for elderly demented patients:

- diagnostic facilities,
- medical and paramedical care,
- evaluation and counselling in collaboration with the social service organizations,
- maintaining the patient's health and well-being and providing rehabilitation (physical medicine, physiotherapy, speech therapy, etc.).

The aims and resources vary greatly from one establishment to another. Some are technically very well equipped.

Basically, day centres watch over the patient and offer occupational therapy and psychotherapy. Day centres have three main advantages:

- they improve the patient's quality of life;
- they lend support to the family;
- they often postpone permanent institutionalization.

However, day centres should not be regarded as an alternative to long-stay institutions, since they are really designed for highly selected patients who are not too dependent. They must be near the patient's home, too, as transport is a serious problem and those doing the looking-after are themselves frequently too old to cope with taking the patient to and from the centre. The patient may refuse to get onto the bus or may behave in a dangerous manner on the bus or while getting off. Even when these obstacles are overcome, 1 in 4 patients is unable to adapt to a day centre.

Day hospitals and day centres may help certain selected patients, but are no substitute for a long-stay institution.

Only big towns have day hospitals and day centres

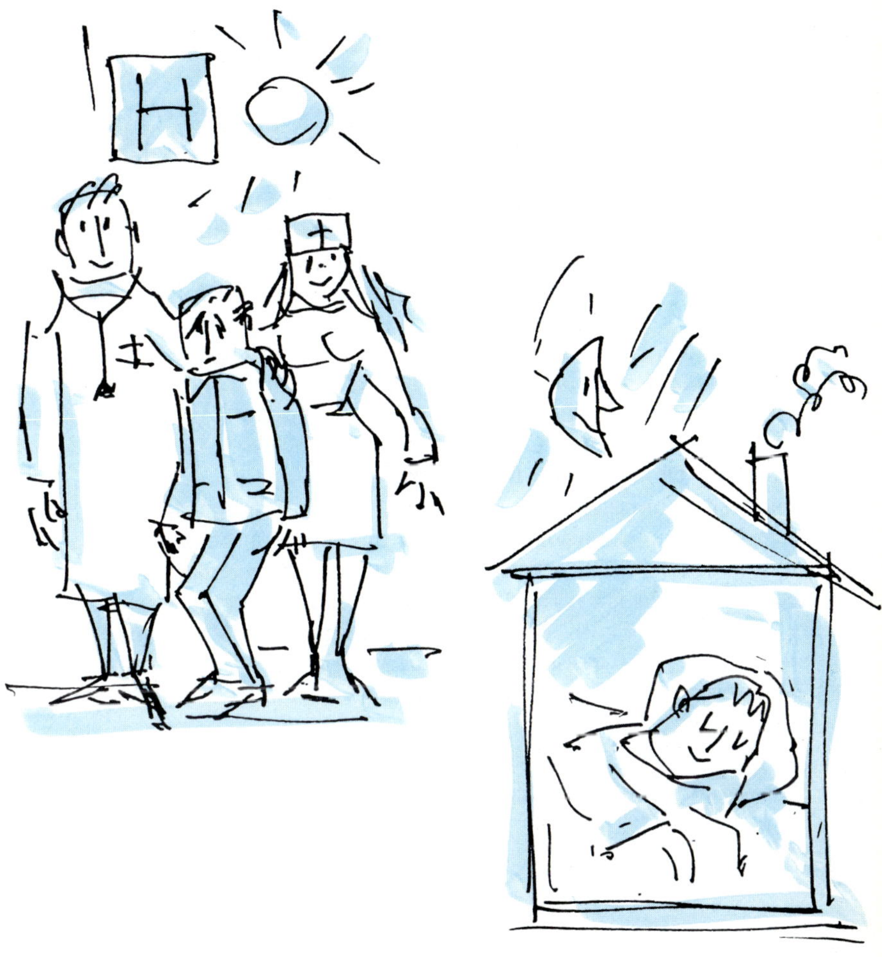

Day hospitals and day centres are suitable only for certain patients who are able to make the journey, are well looked after at home, and who do not life far away.
Patients who are able to take advantage of such an institution normally find a wide range of services. Their families also benefit from the support during the day, which is what they are normally in urgent need of.

The Temporary Hospitalization of the Demented Patient – A Two-Edged Sword

The elderly demented patient may be temporarily hospitalized under three very different sets of circumstances:

(1) *An acute medical or surgical condition* unrelated to the dementia may require his admission to hospital. Many families welcome this unexpected respite and they may try to delay the patient's discharge. *However, the stay in a non-geriatric ward should be as short as possible.* Most hospital wards are not tailored to the needs of this type of patient. The longer the stay in hospital, the less likelihood there is that the patient will return home. The family may ask for the patient to be transferred to an institution, but the circumstances are not propitious unless this has previously been given mature consideration. There is little likelihood that this will be best for the Alzheimer patient.

(2) Those caring for the patient *are unable to cope with particular manifestations of dementia* such as serious behavioural disorders. Temporary admission to an acute ward for the care of elderly demented patients is then desirable, although such facilities are still all too rare. The patient is returned home once the critical period has passed.

(3) Temporary admission may facilitate *rehabilitation after an illness or an operation.* It also gives those looking after the patient a break, enabling them to take a holiday, relax or to undergo medical treatment themselves. The period of hospitalization is fixed on admission. Frequently the staff know the patient, who has been with them before. Temporary hospitalization is a valuable back-up for those caring for the patient at home.

Periods of hospitalization for disorders other than the dementia should be kept to a minimum. Temporary admission to a geriatric ward gives families a welcome break and helps to ensure that the patient can be cared for at home.

Temporary hospitalization must presuppose that the patient will return home

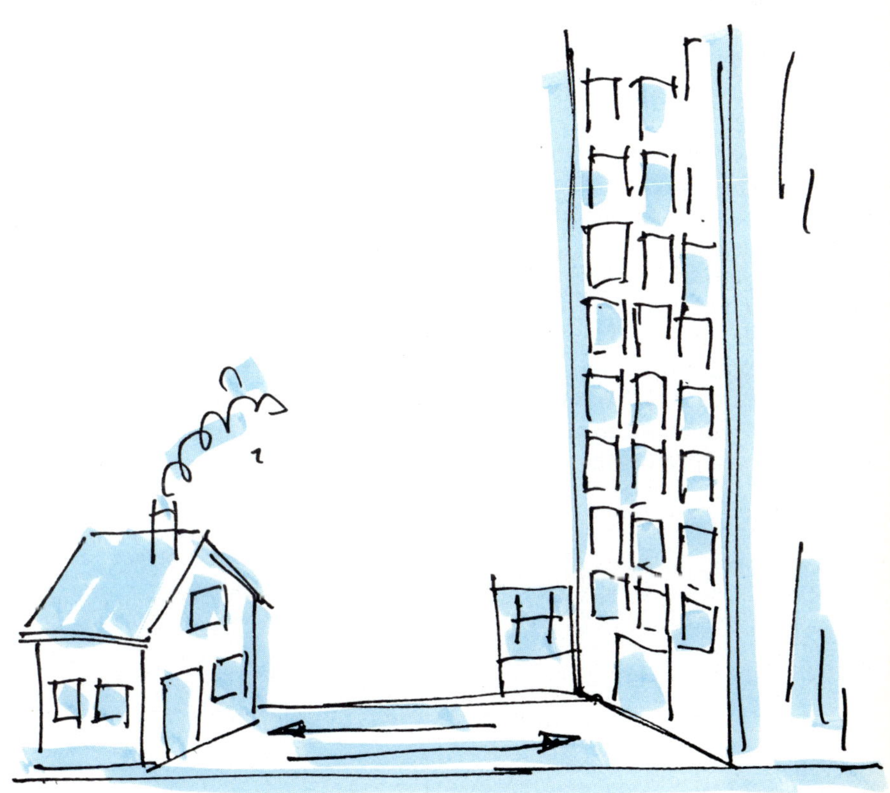

Temporary hospitalization may be necessary for the patient's health and to give the family a break.

The Limitations of Home Care for Demented Patients

Caring for the demented patients at home has long been regarded as the best solution, both for the patient's well-being and from the economic point of view. This is not always the case. In many circumstances admission to an institution is preferable.

Reasons Relating to Patients and Their Environment
Poor housing conditions (cramped quarters, overcrowding, lack of amenities) argue against home care. Some patients require help with all their daily living activities and must constantly be watched day and night. If such services have to be paid for, the cost of keeping the patient at home may outweigh that of institutional care. Also aggressive behavioural disturbances may constitute a danger to the person caring for the patient, in particular if that person is a frail woman with physical disabilities. Mobile patients or those prone to wander may find the restrictions that have to be placed on them for their own safety less irritating in an institution geared to the problem.

Reasons Relating to the Family Circle
Whether or not a patient should be placed in an institution is determined more by the qualities of the persons caring for the patient than by those of the patient himself. Some relatives refuse from the very beginning to care for their demented relative. Others become physically or mentally exhausted after a while and have to give up. In some instances placement in an institution may even protect the patient from ill treatment.

Institutional care is not reserved solely for advanced forms of the disease. It is a better solution than home care where this would be harmful to the patient or his family.

Caring for the patient at home at all costs is not wise

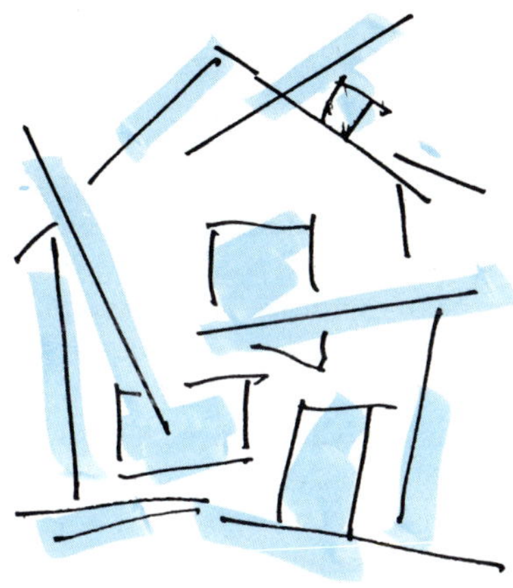

Where living conditions are poor, leaving a demented patient to be cared for in the family is unacceptable for both sides.

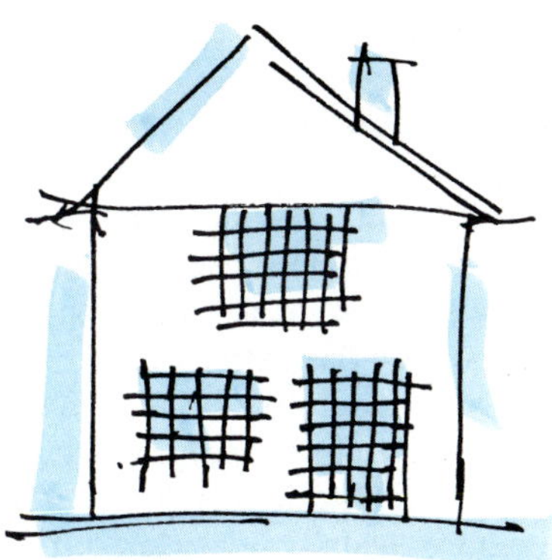

If mobile patients have to be 'barricaded' in a confined space for their safety, transfer to a nursing home is often the better solution for the patient.

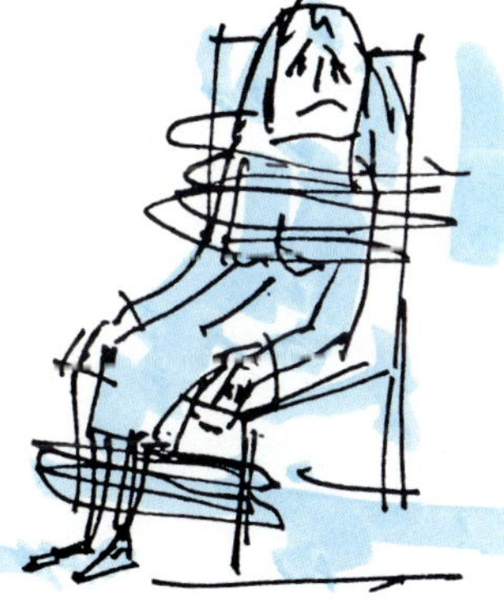

If ordinary measures are insufficient to control behavioural disorders which are dangerous for the patient himself and his family, placement in an institution is indicated.

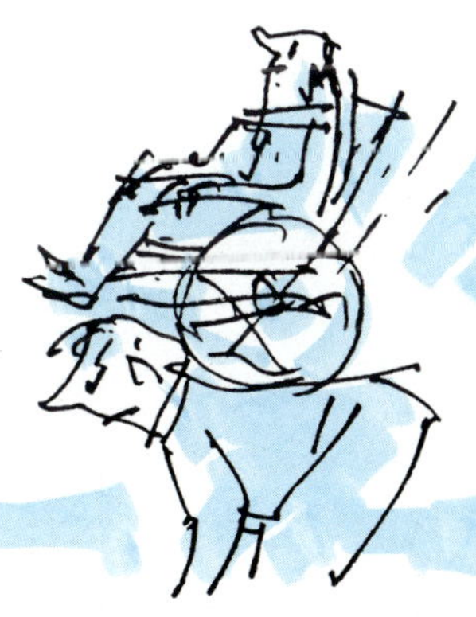

If the burden becomes too great for the person looking after the patient, institutional care is the only way out of the tricky situation.

The Choice of Long-Stay Institution for an Alzheimer Patient

The choice of long-stay institution is a difficult one. Many families refuse even to consider the prospect while they are still able to look after the patient at home. Nevertheless, there comes a time for many patients when they simply have to be admitted to an institution. The choice of institution should therefore *be given some thought by the family at the start of the disease.* Suitable institutions are rare, and the demand is great. The best or most conveniently located institutions have long waiting lists. Fees are high, and social security usually has to contribute. The formalities to be gone through to obtain help with fees usually take several months. Unplanned admission dictated by pressure of circumstances in an emergency situation may well prove disastrous for the patient.

The choice should be based on various criteria, which sometimes clash. The fees, the length of the waiting list, the geographical situation and difficulty of access for the family often rule out an institution from the outset.

The factors usually considered in selecting an appropriate institution are:

(1) *The facilities provided:* the standard of accommodation, the technical equipment, the congeniality of the surroundings, the number of patients for the available space, and the qualification of the staff.

(2) *The service provided:* are the services provided tailored to the needs of the patient? Have the patient's needs been correctly assessed? Are the services provided as and when required?

(3) *Quality of care:* see page 166.

When the condition is first diagnosed, a search must be made for the best institution able to accept the patient, even if it seems unlikely that the patient will ever have to be admitted. The choice is difficult, the formalities are protracted, and the available places none too plentiful.

If it becomes necessary to place an Alzheimer patient in an institution

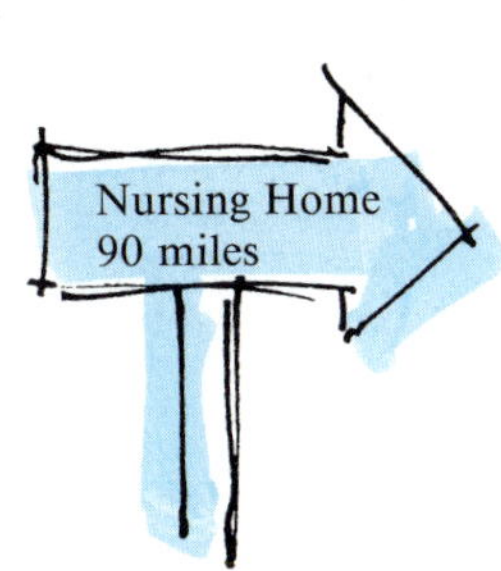

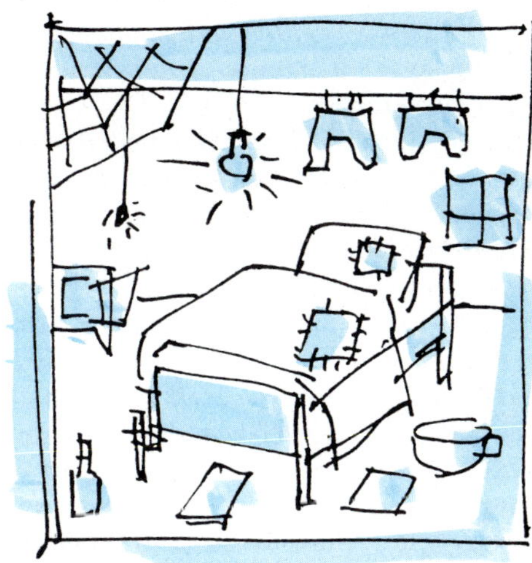

The institution should be fairly near to where the family lives. This is essential where the spouse or child is also elderly. Is public transport available and how frequently do the trains or buses run? How long does the journey take? What is the fare?

Are the rooms well equipped? Are they clean and well maintained?

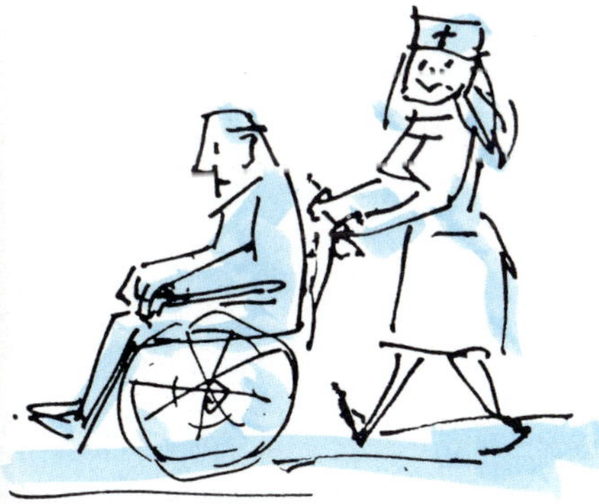

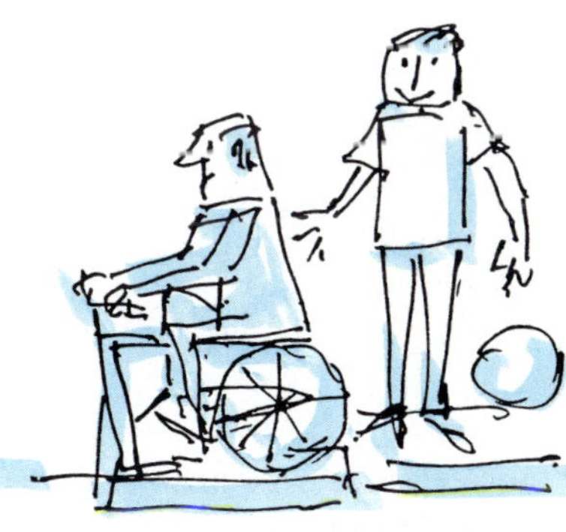

Is staffing adequate both in terms of number and in terms of quality? What services are provided? How are they delivered and by whom?

How to Evaluate the Quality of Care in Long-Stay Institutions

The usual indicators of quality of care cannot be applied in the case of Alzheimer patients (mortality, improvement rate, duration of stay). A useful system based on *negative indicators* has been devised in the USA:

- frequency of incidents of dehydration: these incidents usually indicate poor surveillance;
- changes in weight (unexplained loss of weight or more rarely excessive weight gain); these changes may be observed even in patients who are well looked after but can also result in malnutrition;
- excess use of sedatives;
- frequency of decubitus ulcers;
- routine use of indwelling bladder catheters with no attempt at bladder training;
- excessive use of physical or pharmacological restraints;
- the quality of personal care as evidenced by the condition of the clothing, oral hygiene and the state of the nails and hair;
- prompt response of staff to requests for assistance;
- general cleanliness of the accommodation and materials.

Many complications are sometimes wrongly regarded as inevitable. Close surveillance of patients reduces the frequency and severity of complications. Availability of staff, attention to detail and rejection of easy solutions determine the quality of a long-stay institution.

Long-stay institutions must care for the patient's needs

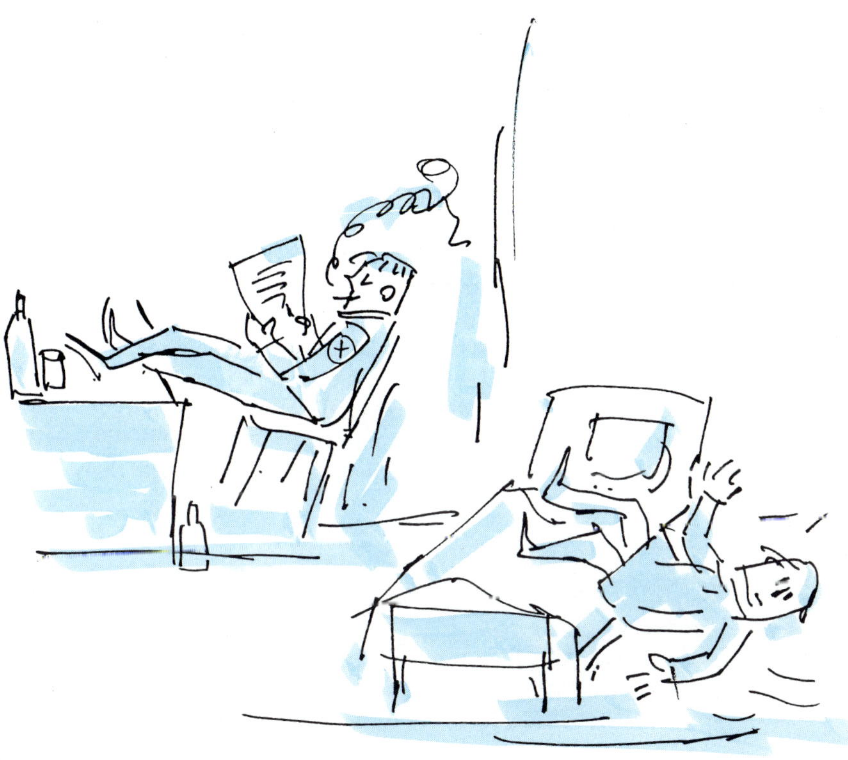

Basically the points which count for most in long-stay institutions are the general atmosphere, the friendliness of the staff, and the well-being of the patients.

What Are the Costs of Senile Dementia?

In Europe and the USA approximately 5% of individuals aged 65 or over are suffering from dementia. This means that there are 300,000 cases in the United Kingdom and a similar number in France. More than two thirds have Alzheimer's disease and one third are suffering from multi-infarct dementia. The cost to society is enormous: it was estimated at 24–48 billion dollars in the United States in 1985. In the United Kingdom the estimated cost in 1976/77 was of the order of £300 million, not including costs borne by families.

In France the cost per day of care in a public long-stay institution in Paris was FFr. 514 in 1988. Social security contributes FFr. 161, leaving FFr. 353 to be met by the patient, i.e. FFr. 10,500 per month. The fees charged by private institutions accepting demented patients vary, but are similar. Most retirement pensions are too small to cover such charges; they are therefore paid by the district welfare organization, which recovers all or part of the sums paid out:

(1) by appropriating the patient's old-age pension, the patient retaining only 10% as 'pocket money';
(2) by mortgaging the patient's property;
(3) by charging children and grandchildren according to their means.

Private insurance schemes are available in the USA and Europe to indemnify relatives who do not qualify for social security. This cover is provided either for persons who may need to be cared for in an institution, or for their children etc. who wish to cover themselves against having to pay for their parents/grandparents.

The cost of dementia is enormous, both to society and to the families involved. The inadequacy of social provisions in some countries has led to the introduction of private insurance schemes to provide relatives with cover for the cost of institutional care for their dependants.

The cost of dementia in different countries

Disease-related minimal monthly costs for long-term care for dementia (costs are calculated without expenses for accommodation, services and food). All values have been adjusted to the cost situation of 1988/89.

	Care within the family		Care at home with domiciliary services (e.g. meals on wheels, laundry service, community nursing etc.)		Institutionalization (basic cost of a nursing home is between SFr. 3,500.– and 5,000.– per month)	
	SFr.	$	SFr.	$	SFr.	$
United Kingdom	149.–	90.00	1,558.–	994.00	1,090.–	660.00
Switzerland	295.–	178.00	1,906.–	1,155.00	1,173.–	727.00
Germany (FRG)	281.–	170.00	1,633.–	989.00	1,373.–	832.00
France	231.–	140.00	1,877.–	1,137.00	1,270.–	769.00
USA	436.–	264.00	1,258.–	968.00	1,556.–	943.00

Exchange rate: SFr. 1 = DM 1.117 = FFr. 3.7813 = £0.3513 = $0.6060.

Numbers of elderly people with senile dementia in various industrialized countries:

	Total number	Living in institutions (20%)	Being cared for at home (80%)
United Kingdom	312,000	61,000	251,000
Germany (FRG)	300,000	60,000	240,000
France	228,000	39,450	188,550
USA	1,800,000	360,000	1,440,000

Caring for a Chronically Demented Patient within the Family

H.P. Wirth

Senile Dementia – Definition and Problems of Diagnosis

Senile dementia is an impairment of intellectual functions that manifests itself as a decline and, ultimately, loss of abilities acquired in earlier years. It has an increasingly detrimental effect on the patient's social, working and family life. Dementia must be distinguished from mental retardation existing from early childhood onwards, which is characterized by the complete non-acquisition of certain abilities, and from intellectual impairment due to single events such as injuries, cerebral infarction, operative brain lesions, etc.

Senile dementia can be due to a number of causes and varies greatly in degree of severity from barely perceptible disability to complete helplessness necessitating constant nursing.

Where possible the term dementia should be qualified by indicating the underlying disorder, since it is used for numerous diseases which, depending on their degree of severity, present in completely different ways. Usually the disease is insidious in onset and initially goes unnoticed. Only with hindsight do relatives realize that changes in the behaviour of the person affected, which they had regarded as transient depression or a sign of normal aging, were in fact the first signs of dementia. This problem is made more difficult by the fact that those affected often do everything they can to cover up their disability. They may react vehemently if their capabilities are called into question and are very reluctant to admit that they are affected, often because they fear the loss of their independence. In addition there is often wide fluctuation in the severity of the signs and symptoms of dementia, especially at the start of the disorder, but also in the later stages, making it more difficult to recognize with certainty.

Senile dementia is a complex psychiatric condition associated with increasing loss of cognitive functions. It may have a variety of underlying causes, while its course is characterized by a slow but persistent deterioration. The nature of the condition itself and the response of those directly and indirectly affected make it difficult to recognize.

Senile dementia – a nightmare for many people

A number of terms are used for conditions characterized by forgetfulness, confusion, impaired orientation and declining mental abilities with advancing age:
- senile dementia,
- Alzheimer's disease,
- cerebral sclerosis,
- chronic cerebral syndrome,
- psycho-organic syndrome (POS),
- organic brain syndrome,
- and many others.

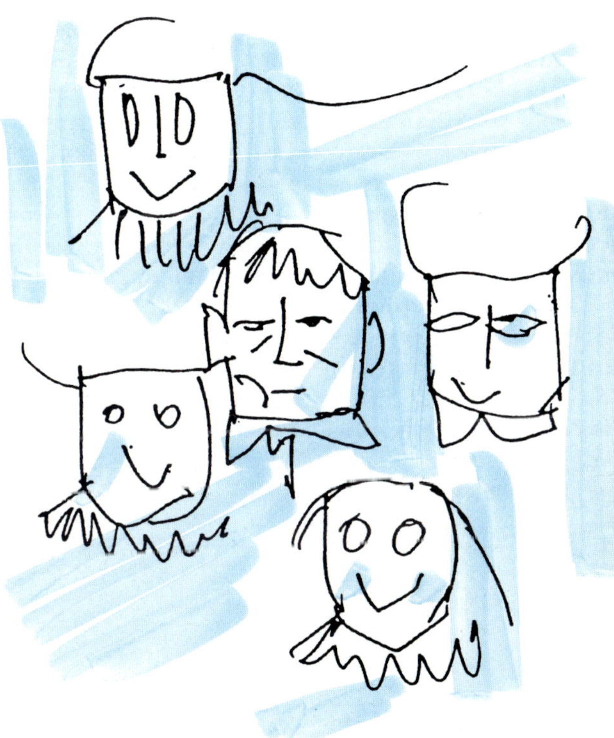

Those affected keep their dementia secret for as long as possible, because dementia is far less socially acceptable than many other diseases. This is also one of the reasons why dementia is coming to be regarded as a psychiatric disorder.

Stages in the Progress of Senile Dementia

In the insidious progression of senile dementia the mental disturbances make their debut in a particular order:

(1) It starts with occasionally forgetting names, failing to keep appointments and losing things. Professional and social activities are not, however, affected.

(2) As the disorder progresses, the forgetting of important appointments becomes more frequent and difficulties are experienced in coping with matters outside the normal routine. However, if stressful tasks are avoided, the symptoms may pass off.

(3) Eventually, however, problems are encountered in doing the shopping, handling money and driving the car. Independence is threatened since bills are either not paid on time or not paid at all.

(4) Help is required in deciding what to wear and personal hygiene is neglected unless it is supervised. Clothes are not put on properly, daytime clothing is pulled on over nightwear, for example, shoelaces and ties are not tied properly and shoes are put on the wrong feet. A simple matter like taking a bath, which involves a succession of acts (going to the bathroom, running the water, adjusting the temperature, undressing, climbing into the bath and washing), appears so complicated that the patient is unable to cope.

(5) There is difficulty in going to the toilet unaided. This is often followed by urinary and then faecal incontinence.

(6) The vocabulary becomes progressively reduced, following difficulty in finding the right words and increasing taciturnity at an early stage. The patient says less and less, ultimately limiting him/herself to a few words.

(7) The ability to walk and stand – and eventually sit – is lost.

Senile dementia typically follows a course in which cognitive defects occur, ranging from serious memory problems to an inability to walk or even stand up.

Patients with full-blown senile dementia lose the ability to communicate

Loss of speech leaves eye movements as the patient's only means of communication. This may be followed by *loss of the ability to chew and swallow,* leading ultimately, if the patient does not succumb to an intercurrent disease, to death.

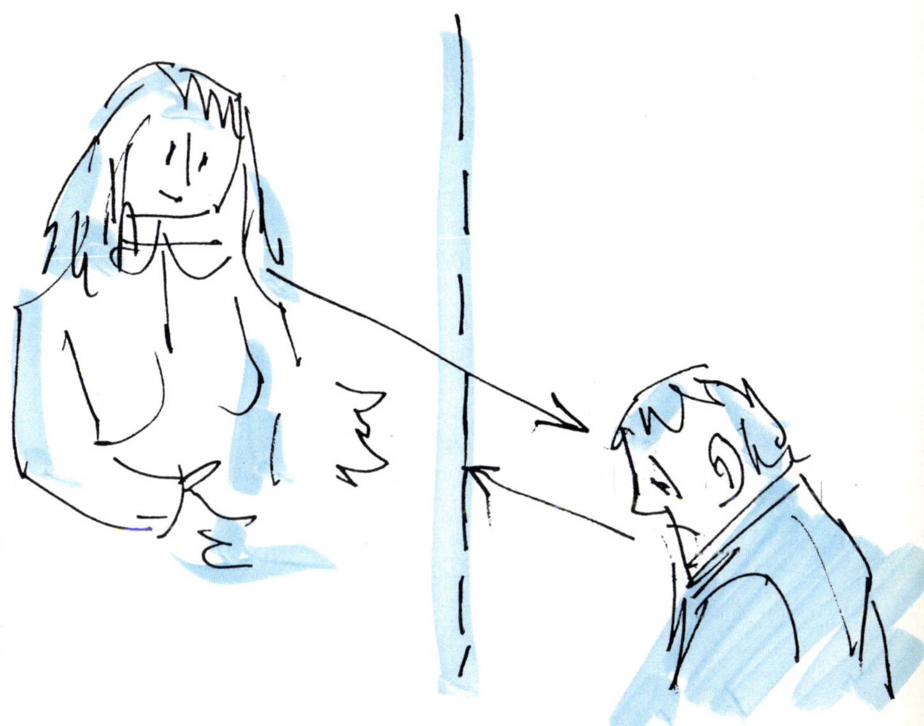

Senile dementia is doubly important, firstly because it is a tragedy for the individual concerned and secondly because of the large numbers involved, with estimates suggesting that 5% of people over 65 years of age are affected. The probability of developing the disorder increases with age so that, with the increasing aging of the population, the numbers of demented individuals are steadily rising. And since it is a progressive disease, most cases require institutional care sooner or later. Places in institutions are expensive and hard to find, however, and it is proving increasingly difficult to recruit suitable staff.

Normal Aging or Early Dementia?

Although it is normal for elderly people to have rather less stamina, to show greater resistance to innovation, and to undergo physical decline, healthy elderly people have their feet firmly rooted in reality and are perfectly capable of leading an independent life. If this is not the case, the possibility of dementia should be borne in mind. Incipient dementia should be suspected if evidence is observed of a striking reduction in energy, a loss of interest in things that used to appear important, of sudden fluctuations in mood and of a constant state of anxiety.

Such people need help, even though they may reject it, but the problem is how to recognize that a person has dementia. Since those in the immediate family circle are generally the first to be aware of subtle changes, it is they who must first take stock of the situation.

The first step is to determine what things the person concerned can still do safely, completely independently and without appreciable mental stress. This assessment must be made very cautiously, ideally without the 'patient' being aware of it. Relatives should always bear in mind that the condition may perhaps be due to a disorder which can, and should, be treated as soon as possible. This is only feasible, however, if they are perceptive enough to recognize that something is amiss. The doctor, too, must rely for his assessment on what the relatives have to tell him, since those affected are seldom able or willing to report impairments of their own performance, preferring to keep them secret, cover them up, or deny them. These are further reasons why the first move must come from those close to the patient.

There is no clear dividing line between normal aging and the first signs of dementia. Early recognition requires careful observation. A departure from, or abandonment of, habits or interests of many years' standing is often an early sign of incipient dementia.

Early senile dementia and normal aging are difficult to distinguish

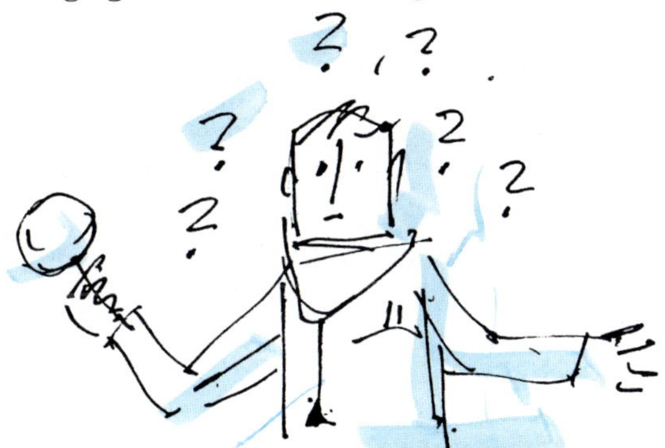

Knowledge of what is normal and what is morbid in elderly people is imperfect. It is important to ensure that a person with suspected impaired mental function is given a sympathetic but nevertheless critical assessment. It should be realized that such an assessment has to be made out of care and affection and not out of a resentful desire to do the person down.

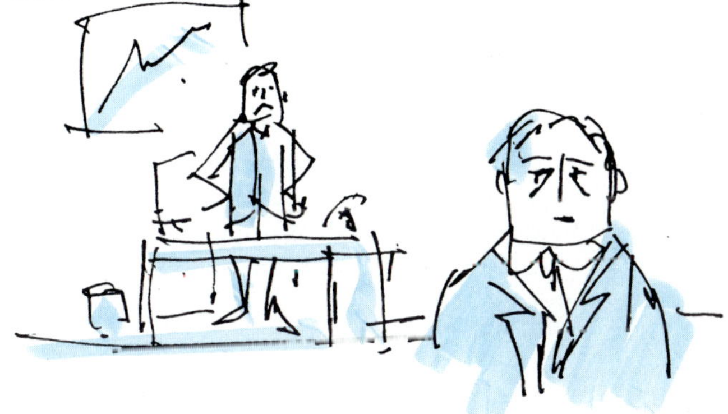

Objective assessment is often somewhat simpler if the problem of impaired mental performance first comes to light through some external event. This is usually an incident such as one of the following:

- The employer indicates that he is dissatisfied with the person's work.
- The family is suddenly confronted with a mountain of unpaid bills or the consequences of senseless business dealings.
- The patient is involved in a road accident.
- The patient suddenly becomes confused as a result of an illness or operation.

Driving a Car and Living Alone – Two Problem Areas in Early Senile Dementia

Driving a Car

Close relatives of an elderly person must take action when that person can no longer drive safely but does not realize if. If the person concerned has been driving for many years without an accident, the readjustment will be particularly difficult.

It is important to look out for warning signs. On noticing a decline in driving skills, action must be taken at once. This requires a sensitive approach. For most people, giving up driving involves an appreciable loss of independence and self-esteem. They may recognize that they are unsure of themselves at the wheel but cannot bring themselves to admit it. Things can be made easier by someone else offering to drive on the pretext, say, of enabling the elderly person to enjoy the countryside in comfort and relaxation. One might also suggest taking the train for similar reasons. If this falls on deaf ears, the doctor may prove more persuasive but, if all else fails, the car keys must be confiscated or the car immobilized by removing the distributor cap, even if this means calling in a car mechanic. Accident prevention justifies even such drastic measures!

It should also be remembered that the aging brain is less tolerant of alcohol, even small amounts of which can diminish self-control in elderly people.

Living Alone

In deciding whether an elderly person can continue to live on his/her own or not, it is best to assume that deterioration will continue and to plan accordingly. Ideally, recourse may be had initially to ways of bridging the gap, e.g. by calling on services such as 'meals on wheels', a home help, the district nurse, etc., and by paying regular social calls.

The ability to go on driving and living alone are two of the most reliable criteria for assessing whether the person concerned has early-stage dementia or not.

Driving and living alone as everyday psychogeriatric test situations

Driving

Principal prerequisites for good driving:

- optimum co-ordination of movements;
- adequate vision and hearing;
- quick reactions;
- alertness;
- decisiveness.

Warning signs of early senile dementia:

- slow or inappropriate reactions;
- steady decline in handling skills;
- ignoring of road signs or markings;
- agitatation, confusion and/or freezing when confronted with an unaccustomed situation;
- loss of orientation in well-known surroundings;
- sudden braking or acceleration without good reason.

Living alone

Old people can no longer be allowed to live alone if the following situations and/or patterns of behaviour occur:

- failure to eat regularly (loss of weight);
- failure to take medication as prescribed;
- poor personal hygiene and domestic cleanliness;
- failure to heat the home in cold weather;
- increasing carelessness in the handling of fire and electrical appliances;
- uncritical trust or distrust of both acquaintances and strangers;
- persecution complexes.

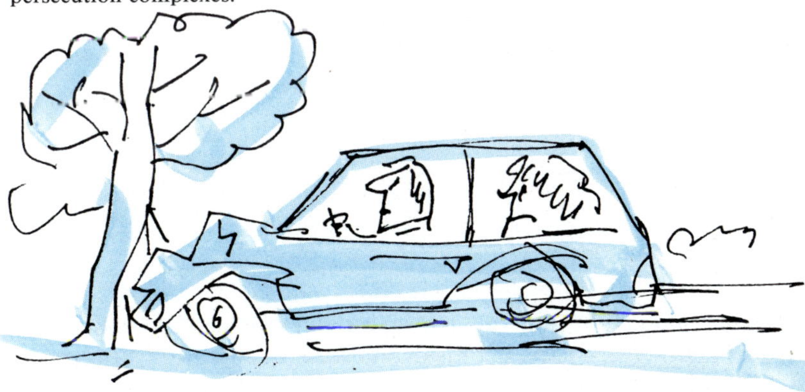

Undertaking to Care for a Demented Patient – How to Approach Such a Decision

If one's family or circle of friends is confronted with the problem of having to care for a demented person, or one has to give advice in such a situation, a number of questions and decisions have to be considered:

Firstly, every action must be carefully thought through in advance. Care should be taken not to rush into giving well-intentioned undertakings that one subsequently finds one cannot keep.

Decisions should not be taken by any one person but should first be discussed in the family. One should consider whether the action or measures decided on are the result of one's own convictions or of pressures from outside. Feelings of guilt are a poor starting point!

The first thing is to be clear about the diagnosis. This involves consulting the doctor, who should be informed of the decision to look after the patient at home. The doctor should also be questioned about the extent of the handicap, possible treatments and the course the disease is likely to follow. It can be a help to note down the most important questions in advance in preparation for such a consultation so that nothing is overlooked. A discussion along these lines can also help to secure the doctor's assistance for the future, should this be required.

Anyone undertaking to care for a demented patient must be prepared for a long and gruelling task and it is advisable to begin looking around from the start for ways of lessening the burden. By no means the least important question is whether one feels physically and mentally up to the task. It is advisable to discuss these points with the doctor, especially as he will probably become the patient's doctor too. He should, by the way, obtain the patient's medical records from his/her previous doctor so as to be fully informed about the patient's medical history.

Assuming responsibility for the care of a demented person should only be undertaken after very careful consideration. It is important to plan things well in advance. No one is indispensable.

Points to be considered when deciding whether to take on the care of a person with dementia

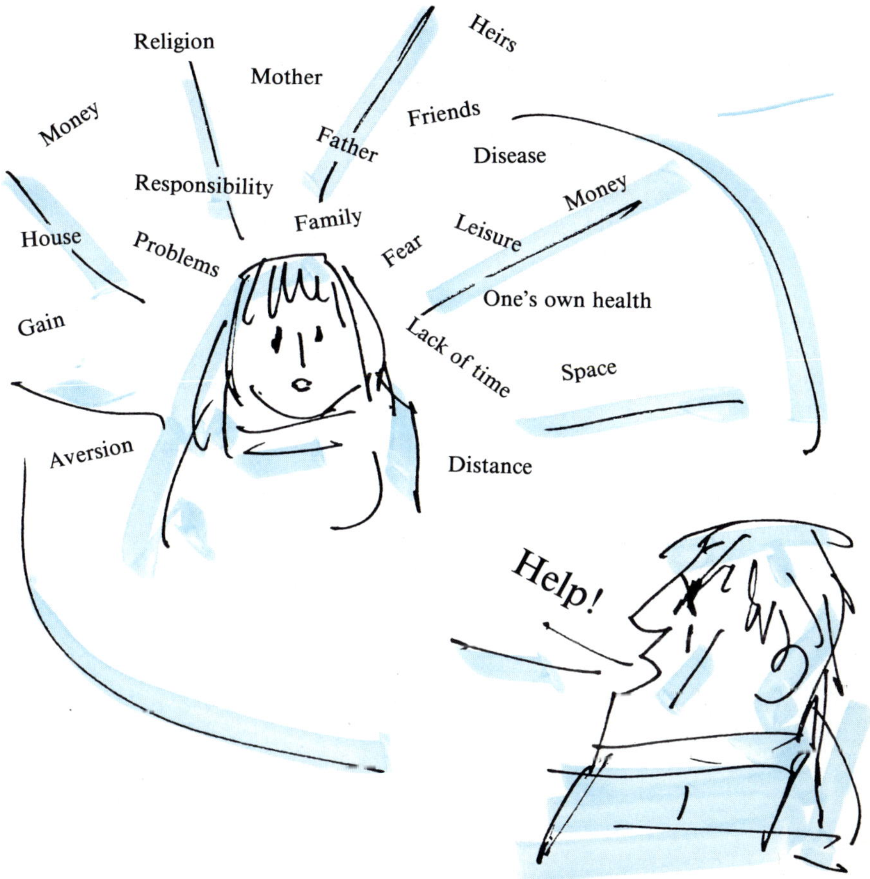

Thoughts such as these, which are likely to come to mind when considering the possibility of caring for a demented patient, should not deter one but should rather serve to prepare the ground so as to ensure a good start. If there are fundamental difficulties, however, they must be taken seriously and solutions found, since measures once decided upon must be persevered with for a time. Unnecessary changes in a demented person's environment must be avoided, since they almost always lead to a deterioration in the patient's condition.

Some Tips for People Taking on the Care of a Demented Relative

When a close relative or one's spouse develops senile dementia, situations may arise which leave no room at all for independent decisions. In the case of a wife or husband, it is usually taken for granted that the 'healthy' partner will care for the patient.

Whenever decisions have to be taken it is vital to keep a cool head, even though all manner of difficulties appear to be looming up at the same time. In such a situation it may make things easier to list the most urgent problems in a notebook in order of priority, breaking complex matters down into more manageable components. Most problems arise from the fact that there are many things the patient is no longer able to do and which have to be done for him. These can often be overcome by simplifying matters and imposing limits.

Problems should always be discussed with relatives and close friends. Though many things might appear trivial to outsiders, this should not deter one from asking for useful suggestions. It is particularly valuable to exchange ideas with other people who are in the same situation, and social security offices can often provide the addresses of self-help groups for relatives of senile dementia patients.

Such groups are usually a source of extremely useful ideas and one can exchange addresses and tips with other members. The greatest benefit of all, however, is the realization that one is not alone with one's difficulties.

A person suddenly confronted with having to care for a patient with senile dementia is often panic-stricken. However, a common-sense approach to the situation and its demands is usually all that is needed – and is certainly much better than bewailing one's lack of nursing training!

Coping with the sudden burden of having to care for a demented patient

Only if one panics will the problems appear insoluble. By drawing up a list of priorities, however, it is always possible to clarify confused situations and arrive at an acceptable solution.

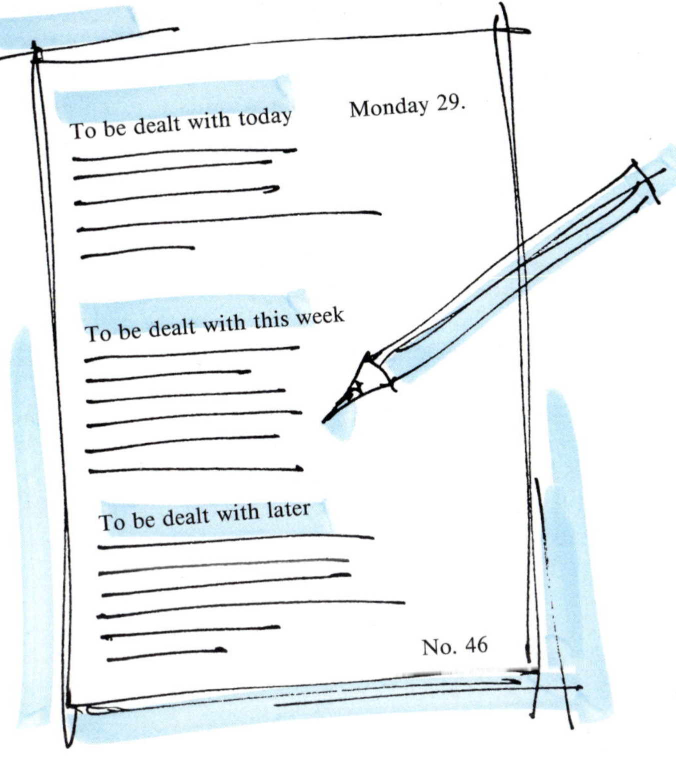

There are limits to what one can do alone and one must be prepared to accept help. Solutions can often be found by asking others how they cope with the same problem, while many difficulties can only be solved in a group. People to whom one can turn for help and advice include one's family, neighbours and acquaintances, the district nurse, the social services, doctors, etc.

Pride should never be a reason for not seeking help! Optimum care can only be achieved through a joint effort.

Detachment Is Needed in Caring for a Patient with Senile Dementia

The patient will often prove irritating, and one may even at times feel hate. Nevertheless, one should not be driven by feelings of guilt to press on grimly with the task in hand. If such a situation arises, it is usually a sign that one is physically and emotionally drained. The best solution in such circumstances is to allow oneself the luxury of a holiday.

Short-lived bouts of irritation can be overcome by reminding oneself of the nature of senile dementia. It is important to remember that the patient has lost control over his or her behaviour, even though he/she may appear to be merely stubborn, indifferent or mischievous. This is often difficult for outsiders to understand, since demented people, externally at least, often appear to be in perfect health, and a few words of explanation can help to avoid embarrassing situations in public.

Once the diagnosis is confirmed, there is no sense in clinging to unjustified hopes. One must face up to the fact that sooner or later the patient will have to be cared for in a home, no matter how fond one is of him/her and how difficult it is to contemplate such a step. This being the case, enquiries should be made at an early stage about waiting times for places in nursing homes.

Obviously one has to adjust one's daily schedule to the needs of the patient, but in so doing one should not neglect one's own needs. If the patient is restless during the night, it is worth taking a nap during the day when the patient does. One should never relinquish valued hobbies and contacts: carers who wear themselves out in a few weeks are benefiting neither themselves nor their 'charges'.

Caring for a patient with senile dementia imposes an enormous mental strain. One should do whatever needs doing in moderation, therefore. Unthinking zeal does more harm than good.

In the long term a patient with dementia can only be helped if the carer preserves the right degree of mental detachment

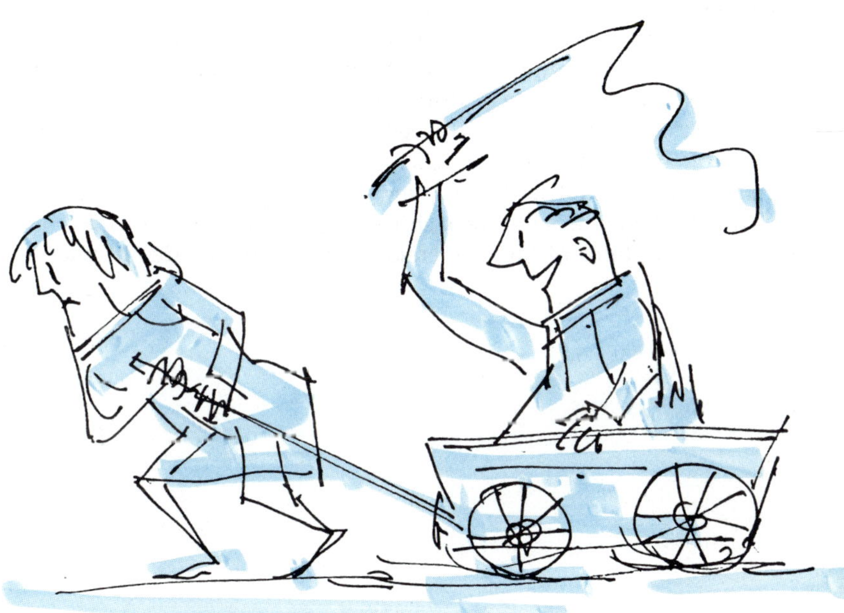

Agreeing to care for a patient does not mean becoming the patient's slave.

General Guidelines for the Day-to-Day Care of Patients with Senile Dementia

First Priorities

Although every case is different and every patient has his or her own particular needs and problems, there are common features, and it is taking advantage of these that makes caring for a demented person tolerable.

A basic requirement is that the carer should have sufficient time for recuperation. One must also be able to take short holidays, which means arranging for relief in good time or finding some other way of bridging the gap. Pangs of conscience at 'deserting one's post', are quite out of place. One can only give adequate care if one feels properly rested, so that ultimately the well-being of the carer also benefits the patient.

Another essential when caring for a patient with senile dementia is to retain one's sense of humour. The ability to laugh at comical happenings is a good sign that the proper detachment is being maintained.

It is also important to make things as uncomplicated as possible. Do only what is absolutely necessary. Perfectionism is counterproductive.

Keep to a timetable. The daily routine should provide stimulation for the patient by constantly requiring his/her co-operation – though without, of course, making excessive demands. It is important that the patient should feel needed and able to participate.

Loss of skills is an inevitable accompaniment of senile dementia, and there is no point in indulging in self-reproach. Stubbornness, maliciousness and moodiness are symptoms of the helplessness engendered by the disease.

Personal care tailored to the patient's particular strengths and weaknesses is important in day-to-day dealings with a demented patient. The loss of skills must be accepted since this is part and parcel of the disease.

A cool head and a warm heart offer the best prospects for successful care

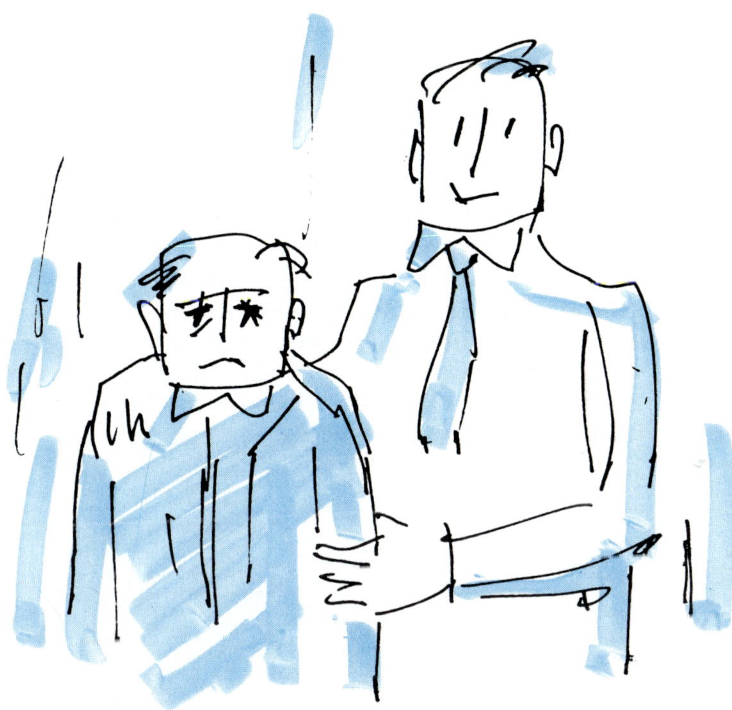

Severely demented people are not particularly attractive, although they are in fact comparable with 1- to 2-year-old children. The disease follows a protracted course (usually over 6–10 years) and is practically unresponsive to treatment, while care is time-consuming and both physically and mentally exhausting. Its worst feature, however, is the sense of hopelessness. Nevertheless, one can have happy times with demented people and feel affection and love for them. Many problems do not really exist – we make them for ourselves or imagine them.

Memory Aids, Verbal Communication and a Timetable Are a Help in Coping with Patients with Dementia

If the patient has lost the ability to understand the written word, simple drawings can be a big help. A metal tag engraved with the name and address and worn round the neck or as a bracelet is extremely useful for patients who run away and wander about in the neighbourhood.

Another typical feature of dementia is lability of mood, with outbursts of emotion that may well be 'over the top' suddenly giving way to outbursts of temper. In this situation it is a help to limit the impressions to which the patient is exposed. The best policy is diversion; do not try to argue. Self-control is important for one's own peace of mind, for the patient will forget the incident far more quickly than you will.

One must speak slowly, loudly and clearly, avoiding involved sentences. Not more than one question at a time should be put to the patient. Moreover, plenty of time must be allowed for an answer. Patients who lose the ability to understand speech continue for a long time to 'understand' gestures of love and affection, despite being severely confused.

The daily routine must be centred on the patient, whose 'performance' often varies considerably over the day. Difficult tasks which have to be performed daily must be scheduled for a time of day when the patient is most responsive. The evening should be a time of tranquillity and rest, although behavioural difficulties often worsen towards evening. Familiar activities in a peaceful environment serve to counteract this tendency.

The gradual loss of memory and the lability of mood call for patience and firmness. The patient's idiosyncrasies should be respected, provided this does not hinder the process of caring for him. However, one must definitely avoid disregarding one's own needs.

Dementia involves increasing loss of memory

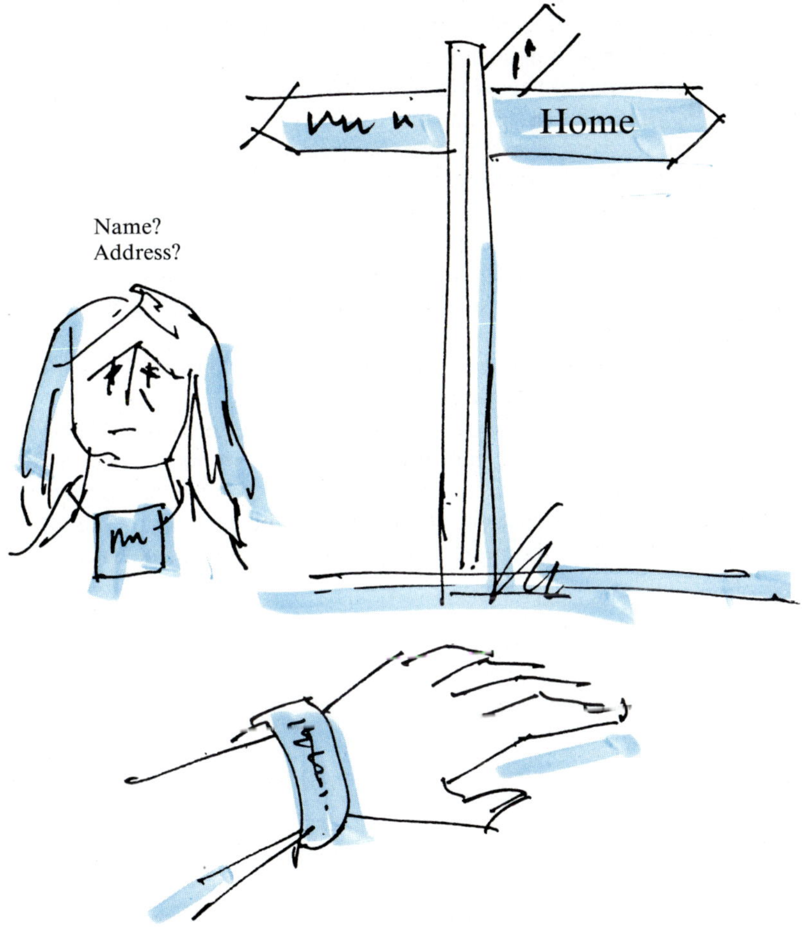

Loss of memory reaches the point where the patient can no longer remember his/her name and address. This can be a major problem in cases where there is a pathological urge to run away or to wander about at night.

The Importance of Accident Prevention Measures with Elderly Demented Patients

The increased accident proneness of demented patients arises from impairment of gait and balance, increased forgetfulness and, by no means least, impaired judgement. Hence an environment has to be provided which takes into account the needs of the patient, not only in terms of equipment and installations, but also of atmosphere because accidents occur more frequently where there is tension and agitation.

The following tips will help to avoid accidents:

A tidy place is generally safer than an untidy one! Potentially dangerous equipment such as irons, bread slicers, hairdriers, sewing machines, lawnmowers, etc. should be removed. Keys, especially car keys, should not be left lying around.

Thought should also be given to the patient's steadiness when standing or walking. Put yourself in the patient's position as you walk around, looking out for potential hazards which might lead to scalding, burns or fires. These must be removed.

If the patient smokes, this should only be allowed under supervision – though it is safer, of course, to give up smoking altogether.

The patient's impaired judgement should also be borne in mind. For this reason, all drugs and household chemicals should be kept under lock and key. Needles, buttons and other small objects should be removed, since they may be swallowed. Poisonous house plants should also be removed. Glass doors should be marked so as to be more easily visible to reduce the risk of collisions.

Depending on the degree of severity of their disease, patients with senile dementia are very prone to accidents. As a result, household objects which are otherwise perfectly safe can become sources of danger.

Accident prevention precautions that a person caring for a senile dementia patient should take

The following measures reduce the risk of a senile dementia patient having an accident in the home:

- Non-slip carpets should be fitted.
- Stair carpet fittings should be checked.
- Raised carpet edges should be fastened down.
- Slippery floors should be fitted with non-slip coverings.
- Handrails on stairs must be checked to ensure that they are not loose.
- Gates or extra rails should be fitted at the top of the stairs.
- Articles with sharp edges should be removed.
- Breakable objects should be put in a safe place.
- Windows should be secured.

Potential hazards which might lead to scalds or burns should be eliminated:

- Hot water taps should be clearly marked.
- The boiler temperature should be set as low as possible to avoid scalds.
- Entrances to the heating system and boiler should be locked.
- Cookers and ovens should be secured by an additional, hidden main switch.
- Smokers' requisites should not be left lying around.

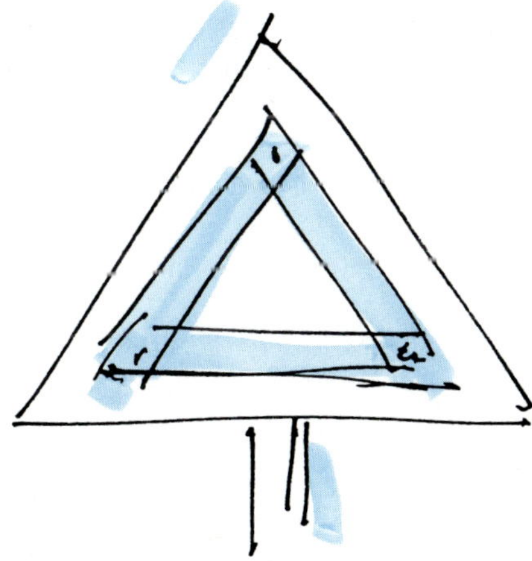

Once the disease has progressed to a certain point, demented patients can no longer ensure their own safety. For this reason, the same precautions must be taken as taken by parents of young children – namely, removal of all possible hazards.

Feeding a Senile Dementia Patient – A Problem in Its Own Right

Ensuring an adequate diet may be fraught with unforeseen difficulties and it is useful to enquire of the appropriate health and social services what help is available to facilitate the task. In many places organizations exist which deliver meals to the home ('Meals on Wheels Services') and any acquaintances who make use of this service should be asked for details. Another possibility is take-away food, which is available from many restaurants.

Confused people may forget about food altogether, even when it is put in front of them. They often throw food away or hide it, and eat it later when it has gone bad. Sometimes patients develop strong aversions to or preferences for certain foods and this can lead to malnutrition. If proper eating cannot be guaranteed, the doctor should be asked to prescribe vitamin and trace element supplements.

Poorly fitting dentures should be corrected by a dentist. Care should also be taken that food is not too hot to eat. It is important that mealtimes be punctual, otherwise the patient may become excessively agitated.

One needs to be tolerant where eating habits are concerned and to realize that a demented patient cannot be forced to eat nicely. Meals should always be taken in a calm and relaxed atmosphere.

Demented patients sometimes forget to chew their food. If food should enter the airways, the patient is no longer able to speak, cough or breathe, and turns blue in the face. If this happens, help must be given at once, or it will be too late: grasp the patient firmly below the ribs from behind and squeeze with both arms in a series of jerks. The resultant pressure wave should dislodge the foreign body from the larynx. It should be remembered that patients often swallow dentures and this can lead to suffocation.

Many problems are encountered in feeding senile dementia patients, ranging from 'messy' eating habits to complete inability to eat.

The senile dementia patient needs additional help in coping with mealtimes

Some tips on the subject of mealtimes:

- Tablecloths and tablemats which can be wiped clean are very practical.
- A bib is useful so that the patient does not 'dribble' food onto his clothing.
- The business of eating should be kept simple by serving one item at a time together with the appropriate eating utensils.
- Cutlery with large handles is easier to manage.
- Heavy cutlery helps the patient to realize that he/she has something in his/her hands.
- Dishes should be placed on non-slip mats.
- Unbreakable plates and dishes should be used.
- If the patient has difficulty in drinking, a feeding cup could be used.
- For patients who have difficulty in chewing and swallowing, food should be cut up small.

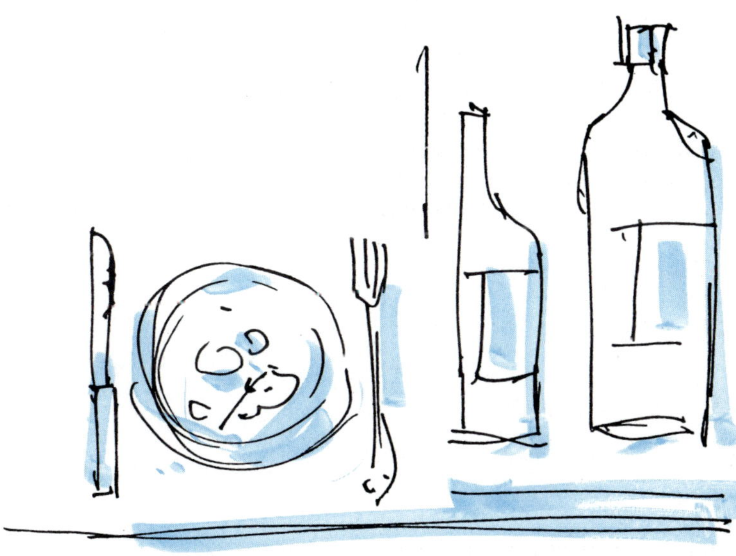

The fork should, of course, be on the left – but no perfectionism, please!

What to Do if a Senile Dementia Patient Stops Eating

The patient's weight should be checked regularly. A sudden loss of weight may be due to an intercurrent disease. To be on the safe side, the doctor should be consulted.

Sometimes a patient can be coaxed into resuming eating by persuasion or by bribery with a favourite dish. If the problem becomes so acute that the only possibility left is feeding by stomach tube, all those concerned for his welfare must be consulted about whether or not this and/or other measures are desirable. This is one of the most difficult of all decisions and should be taken in consultation with the family doctor. The following are some of the points that should be considered:

- Any wishes previously expressed by the patient should be respected, taking account of the new overall situation.
- If the patient pulls the stomach tube out, this is not to be interpreted necessarily as a definite indication of intent.
- If the patient refuses to drink, this does not necessarily mean that he or she is rejecting all help. Old people feel less thirst than younger people and unwillingness to drink is primarily a sign of not feeling thirsty. The danger of dehydration should, however, be borne in mind.
- Is the refusal of food due to a temporary unwillingness or to a permanent inability?
- The additional stress factor of any measures decided on must be weighed against the expected benefit.
- No decision is irrevocable and reassessment may be necessary at any time.

Patients who can no longer swallow and are thus unable to eat or drink always present a difficult problem, even for those who are frequently confronted with this situation professionally. The solution will ultimately depend on the particular circumstances of the situation.

Artificial feeding – yes or no?

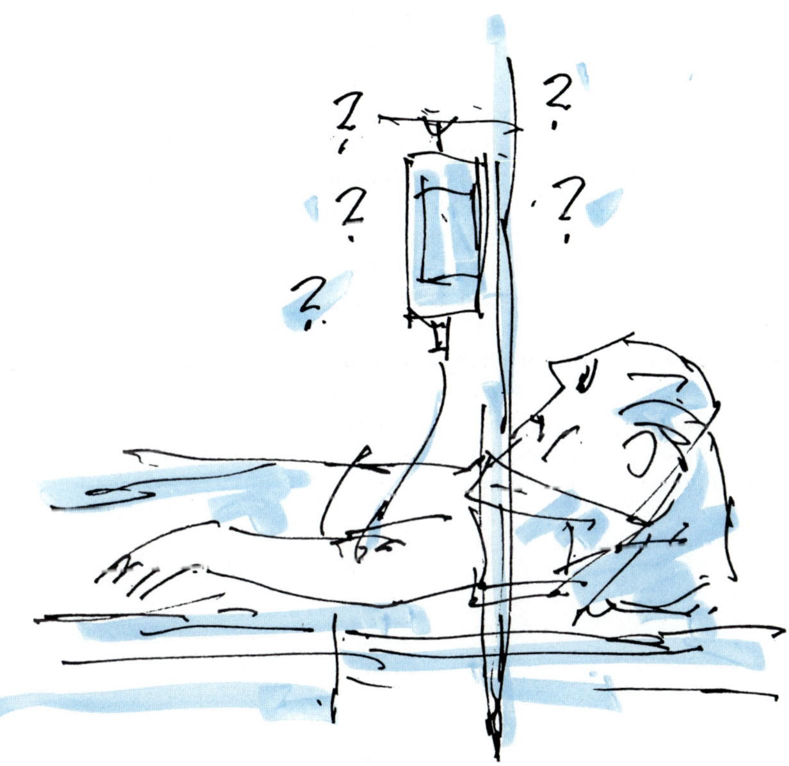

There are no hard and fast rules for deciding whether a patient should be fed by enteral nutrition, and if so for how long. Ultimately it is a matter of judgement based on the particular circumstances of the case.

The Problem of Drug Regimens in Patients with Senile Dementia

If drugs have to be prescribed, the following details must be requested from the doctor:

- What drugs have to be taken?
- What dosage must be taken and when?
- What are the various drugs for?
- What are the principal side effects?

Dementia patients frequently keep drugs which are long past their expiry date – and even take them! For this reason, medicines that have passed the expiry date and any whose age is not determinable should be discarded.

Even if the patient is still basically capable of taking drugs unsupervised, a check should nevertheless be made from time to time. Usually it will be necessary for someone to put the patient's 'pills' out so they are not forgotten, and special plastic boxes are available with separate compartments for morning, midday and evening of each day of the week. This device greatly increases drug compliance and is particularly useful if one is also taking medication oneself. Care must be taken that the patient does not take drugs prescribed by different doctors – unless they have conferred with one another.

One must make sure the patient really swallows the tablets etc. he needs and does not simply keep them in his mouth, then spit them out. The problem can be made easier by administering the drugs with a drink. If the patient has difficulty in taking drugs, the doctor should be consulted to choose the best dosage form (e.g. drops). It is also important to ask the pharmacist whether the tablets may be crushed. All drugs should be kept in a safe place to which the confused person has no access.

It is important to know which drugs the patient really needs and then to ensure that these are actually taken. As a general rule, elderly people are prescribed too many drugs.

A simple aid to drug compliance for patients with senile dementia

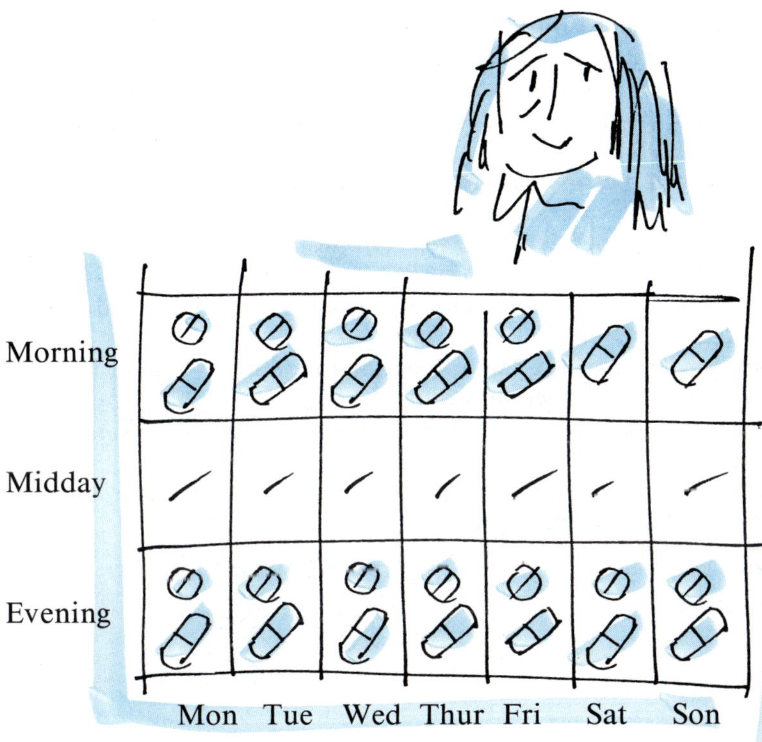

Only drugs which are really necessary should be taken – but then strictly as directed!

Personal Hygiene in Patients with Senile Dementia

Bathing is often fraught with particular problems. Even suggesting that a patient needs a bath can precipitate an angry outburst. Calm and objective explanations do more good than endless arguments. It is a good idea to choose a time of day when the confused person is most lucid, and it is important to follow exactly the same routine each time. Aids such as a shower seat, non-slip mats and mixer taps are a great help. The water temperature must be exactly right and the depth not more than a few centimetres. A confused person must never be left alone in the bath, and bath salts, etc. should not be used since they increase the risk of slipping. The following procedure is recommended: After washing, thorough drying of all parts of the body is important. The skin requires particular attention and areas of skin-to-skin contact should be powdered with talc. Dry skin should be rubbed with plain body oil. The body should also be examined regularly for small injuries and early signs of bedsores.

Relieve the pressure on sensitive areas by ensuring that the patient does not sit or lie in the same position for long periods. Bedsores are particularly prone to develop at points where the skin lies close to the bone (e.g. the sacral region).

The patient's hairstyle should be practical as well as attractive.

Fingernails should be kept short.

Oral hygiene and the care of dentures are important both for the patient's comfort and for proper nutrition.

The ears should be cleaned regularly to prevent impacted wax from impairing hearing.

A high toilet seat is an advantage. Commodes, chamber pots and urine bottles are useful during the night.

Personal hygiene is very much neglected by patients with dementia and requires increasing supervision. Regular checks are necessary to forestall unpleasant surprises, since a person who is confused is incapable of reporting that something is wrong.

The arduous job of supervising a demented patient's personal hygiene

The daily bath calls for great diplomacy on the part of the carer and some measure of mental lucidity on the part of the patient.

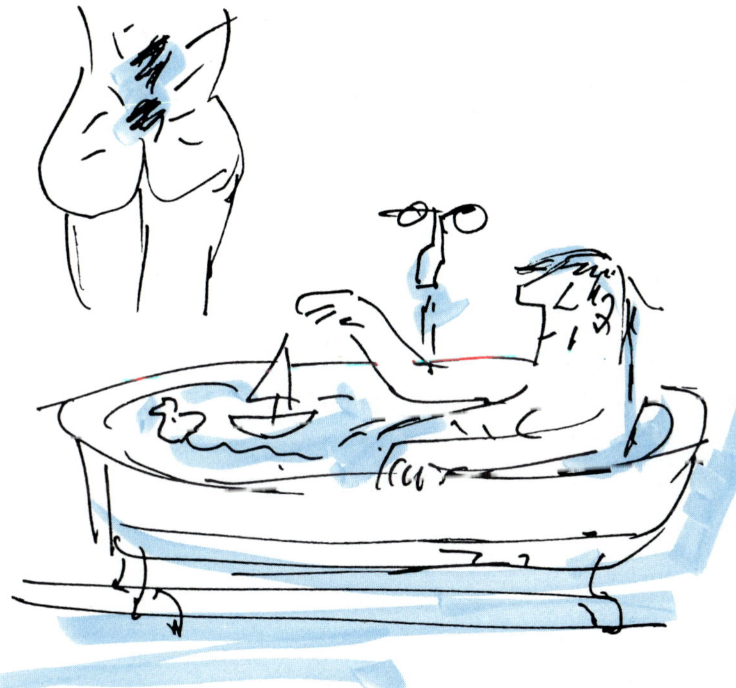

A regular routine for bathing or showering gives the patient confidence and increases his trust in the person looking after him.

Coping with General Medical Problems in Patients with Senile Dementia

Bed-wetting – and even soiling – frequently occurs at some point during the course of the disease. Again, this is due to loss of an acquired ability, namely control over the sphincter muscles. A treatable cause should first be sought, especially if incontinence occurs suddenly and in association with fever. Sometimes the problem is not incontinence at all, but merely an inability to find the toilet or to cope with the clothing.

Bed-wetting can be reduced by redistribution of the patient's fluid intake, leaving a nightlight burning or providing a chamber pot, but it might be necessary to ask the doctor about the possibility of inserting a bladder catheter. Incontinence is not merely an extra burden, it also increases the danger of bedsores developing.

Patients with dementia are more likely to contract other diseases, and these in turn negatively affect their dementia. Sudden deterioration is often due to an infection, a difficulty being that the patient often cannot say exactly what is wrong. If signs and symptoms occur that are not usual for senile dementia, the doctor must be contacted at once.

Not every sign of disease is necessarily a manifestation of the dementia. Like anyone else, patients with dementia can fall victim to other diseases, and these require diagnosis and treatment.

Sudden changes in the patient's condition are probably due to another disorder, unless there is evidence to the contrary

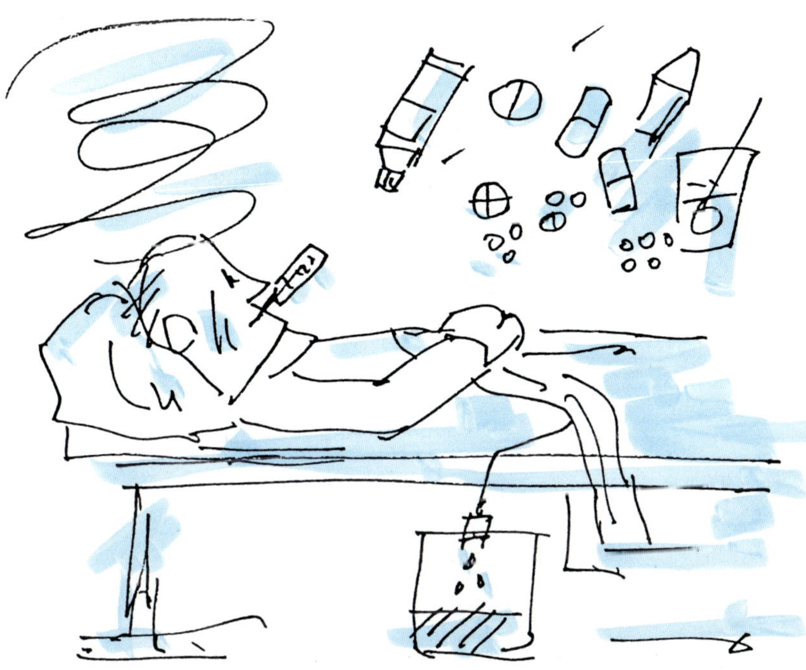

The patient's age alone is a poor excuse for sloppy diagnosis and half-hearted treatment!

However, a supervening illness can be accepted as an act of providence offering relief from a tormented existence, and thus not treated. The ultimate criterion is an assessment of the patient's likely quality of life in the event of recovery, in consultation with all concerned.

Behavioural Disorders in Patients with Senile Dementia

Depending on the severity of the disease, a variety of behavioural disorders may be most prominent:

Impairment and ultimately loss of memory and learning ability: this is an inevitable feature of the disease but is often difficult to understand and accept because the overall impression and the behaviour of the patient in company continue to appear normal.

Running away and wandering about the streets: this is a difficult problem to solve. It can be acute, especially if there has been a change of location, but often passes once the patient has become familiar with the new environment. Changes of domicile should therefore be kept to a minimum and effected gradually so that the patient has sufficient time to accustom himself to new surroundings.

Reversal of the daytime/night-time rhythm with severe inability to sleep at night: any causes that can be discerned should be eliminated if possible.

Mislaying things and accusing others of stealing them: this is due to the typical memory impairment. In the firm conviction of having been robbed, the patient then starts hiding everything, but promptly forgets the hiding place. This reinforces the belief that thieves are at work! One should not take offence at any accusations of this kind, but realize that it is pathological behaviour which the patient cannot control.

Pathological behaviour patterns are often harder to bear than the increasing dependence of the patient, although there are ways of coping. One has to keep telling oneself that behavioural disturbances are simply a feature of senile dementia.

'Sleepless nights' – one of the most difficult things to put up with

Measures which may be taken to combat 'disturbed nights' include:

- Elimination of all potential problems due to having to go to the toilet during the night.
- Provision of a sufficient degree of stimulation during the day.
- Not letting the patient sleep for long periods during the day.
- Exploitation of any familiar objects or habits the patient has which help him to sleep.
- A quiet chat before going to sleep often works wonders.
- A nightlight may overcome the confusion patients feel when they wake during the night.
- Try giving the patient a cup of coffee at bedtime; odd though this may sound, coffee may stimulate the circulation in elderly people and help them fall asleep.
- If all else fails, the doctor should be asked to prescribe a hypnotic or tranquillizer.

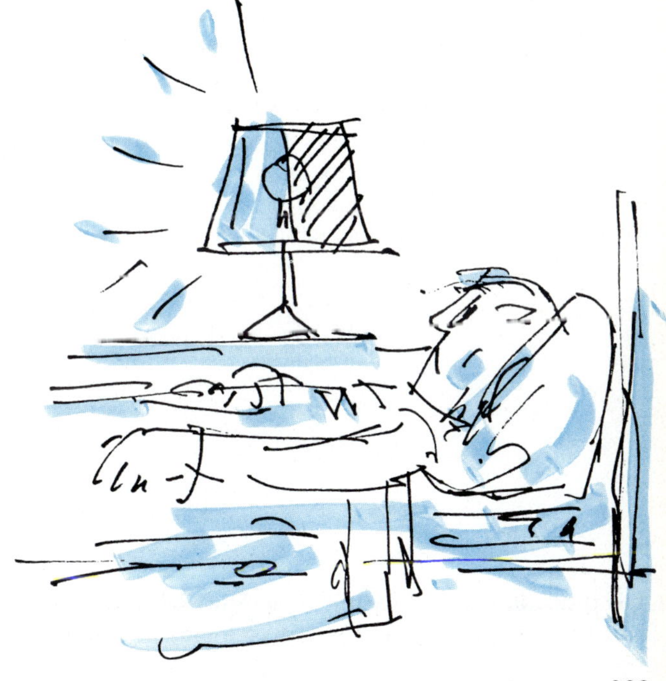

Delusions, Depression and Apathy Are Typical of Patients with Senile Dementia

Patients with senile dementia often tend to keep on asking the same questions, repeating the same actions, making the same accusations, etc. This is a result of the impairment of recent memory, which also has its advantages, however, in that it enables one to divert the patient from his repetitive questioning, etc. Physical activity often provides the best diversion.

Reproaches should not be taken seriously, even though they may be very insulting. Attempts to convince the patient that they are unjustified are in any case pointless. The most effective way of reacting is to close one's ears and let it pass.

Demented people can sometimes become increasingly kind, polite and obliging, showing that it is not only bad character traits that can be exaggerated by the disease.

Some patients develop fixed ideas, hallucinations, increased suspiciousness, delusions, etc. This may be due to misapprehension by the impaired sense organs or to the impairment of recent memory, which leaves intact the memory of people and places long ago but effaces the memory, for example, of the recent death of such a person. Viewed in this way, claims about visits from people who are in fact dead become more understandable. However, a genuine mental disorder may be present if delusional ideas occur that cannot be explained; if such ideas are fairly extreme, drug therapy is needed.

The same applies when there is excessive dejection and apathy, since the transition to genuine depression is a continuum. Depression should in fact always be considered as a possible cause in any case of dementia. A course of treatment with antidepressants is always worthwhile.

The transition between senile dementia and true mental disease is a continuum. Accordingly, psychotropic drug therapy is often necessary.

Dementia may develop into a mental disease

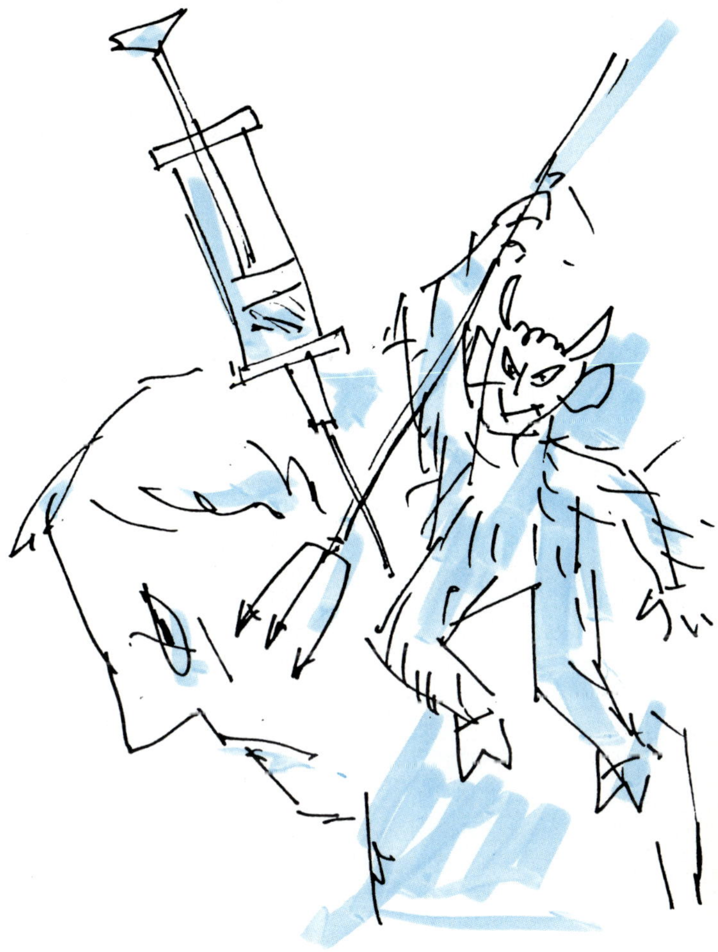

The inappropriate or excessive use of drugs in elderly people can give rise to severe behavioural disorders. On the other hand, some demand specific treatment with drugs, sometimes in high doses for short periods.

Subject Index